# COZY'S COMPLETE
# GUIDE TO GIRLS' HAIR

XOX,

Cozy

# COZY'S COMPLETE
# GUIDE TO GIRLS' HAIR

## COZY FRIEDMAN
*with* SHERYL BERK

ARTISAN
*New York*

*To my mom: Your love, strength,
and determination are inspirational. I love you.*

Published by Artisan
A division of Workman Publishing Company, Inc.
225 Varick Street
New York, NY 10014-4381
www.artisanbooks.com

Published simultaneously in Canada by Thomas Allen & Sons, Limited

Library of Congress Cataloging-in-Publication Data
Friedman, Cozy.
Cozy's complete guide to girls' hair / Cozy Friedman with Sheryl Berk.
p. cm.
ISBN 978-1-57965-422-1
1. Hair—Care and hygiene. 2. Girls—Health and hygiene. 3. Hairstyles.
4. Hairdressing. I. Berk, Sheryl. II. Title. III. Title: Complete guide to girls' hair.
RL91.F75 2011
646.7'24083—dc22
2010033285

Design by Susan E. Baldaserini

Printed in China

5 7 9 10 8 6 4

# Contents

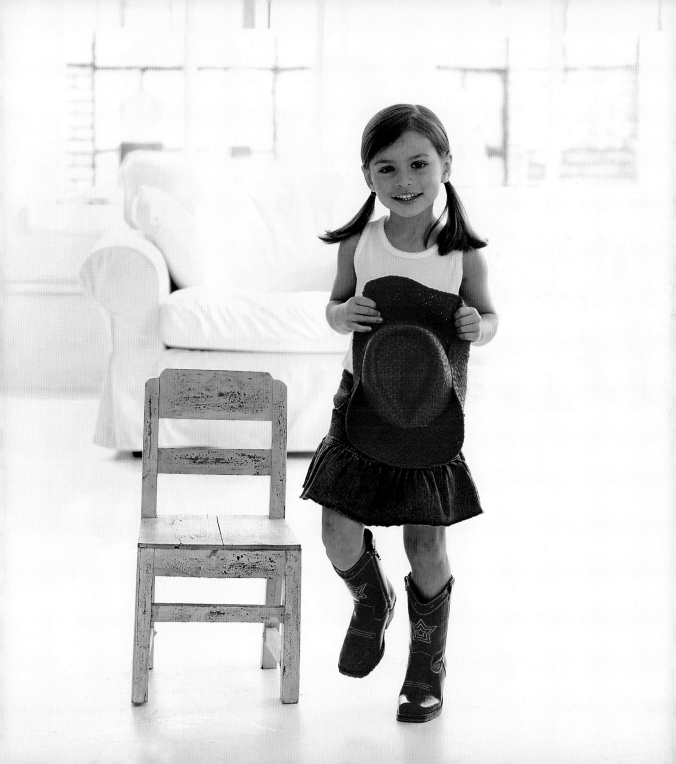

## A Note from Cozy

If someone had told me when I was twelve years old that I would one day be an authority on girls' hair, I would have laughed. As a kid, I had total hair envy. I was born with curly hair, yet I longed to have a straight, bouncy bob like ice skater Dorothy Hamill. No matter how I tried to beat my hair into submission, it never did look like Dorothy's. It took me many, many years to perfect a blowout—but more than that to understand my hair's texture and embrace it. Now I know how to manage my hair so I can wear it curly or straight and be happy either way.

After nearly twenty years of owning Cozy's Cuts for Kids in New York City, I've seen thousands of girls come through my salon's doors. Our clients range from celebrity children and models to "regular kids." Each child is unique, each one looks different, but they all want to feel beautiful and special. Truth be told, hair is a big part of a girl's self-esteem. It is also the ultimate accessory to any outfit; it can convey a mood and celebrate a moment. It can be playful, elegant, even express a child's individuality and personality.

For years, people have been asking me to write a book about girls' hair. Although it seemed like a monumental task to gather all this information, I admit it was an appealing idea. I am the mom of two boys, and I don't get to put my skills and knowledge to use at home! There's a lot of info out there about hair—but it can be confusing and often it doesn't really relate to your child's specific needs.

That's where this book is different. No matter what your child's hair type, length, texture, or issues, you'll find all the answers you need on these pages.

I asked parents what they wanted to know—like how to detangle hair painlessly; how often to wash/condition; and what to do if your child has a hair emergency.

Then I went straight to the source—the girls themselves—and asked what styles they love. Glam girl? Flower child? Fairy princess? Whatever look your little girl is longing for, it's in here. I've compiled our salon's most popular styles—braids, updos, twists, buns, and ponytails—and included step-by-step how-tos. Think of this book as your own private hair tutor!

Even if you have no time to spare, I promise you, your child can have great hair. If your daughter, niece, or granddaughter is in the mood for a new cut (or in awe of some celebrity's new look), simply flip through the pages and you'll find dozens of ideas and easy instructions. I've even included some of my salons' best-kept secrets—like how to cut hair at home, find styles that flatter every face, and choose the right tools and products.

I want girls to feel good about themselves—and I want to empower parents to help their children realize their true beauty, on the inside as well as the outside. When you look good, you feel good; it's as simple as that. This book will help parents to help every girl bring out the best in her hair and herself. Here's to a good hair day and having fun . . . because when you're a girl, that's what hair is all about.

Love,

Cory

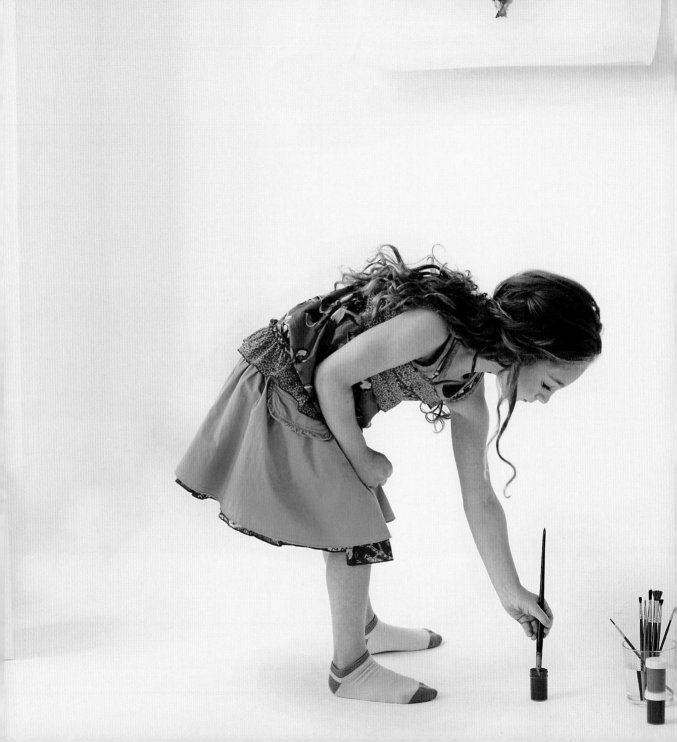

# CHAPTER 1

# A Head Start on Great Hair

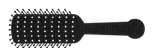

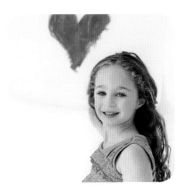

***Girls love hair.*** And why wouldn't they? It's beautiful and magical, and it can be transformed into an endless array of shapes and styles, no fairy godmother required. Just as your child expresses her personality through the clothes she likes or how she keeps her bedroom, her hair is also a mirror of who she is. Sometimes her hairstyle says to the world, "I feel silly"; other times it may proclaim, "I'm a big girl now!" It's fun and liberating for a girl to be able to switch her style—and her persona—with just a few clips, braids, or curls.

Hair has power. Think of how the perfect new cut can make you, as an adult, look and feel ten years younger—or ten pounds thinner. That special feeling goes for any age: The right coif gives you confidence. But no two heads of hair are alike. Your child's hair may be completely different from yours or even her siblings'. It's as unique and special as she is. So, to help her hair become its prettiest and healthiest, you first have to get to know it from the inside out.

## What Is Hair and Where Does It Come From?

Each strand of hair is produced by a hair follicle, a tiny organ that's found just under the skin's surface. Each hair follicle has its own blood supply and nerve endings (that's why if someone pulls your hair, it hurts!). The part of the hair inside the follicle is called the hair root. At the base of the hair root is the hair bulb, where nutrients are received and new cells are formed. The portion you see coming out of the head is the hair shaft, or strand, and it is dead tissue, just like your fingernails, toenails, and the outer layers of your skin. There are no nerve endings in the strand, which is why your hair doesn't feel anything when it's being cut.

Each strand of hair is made up, generally, of three layers.

*The cuticle* is the outer layer of the hair, or "skin" of the hair. Its protective "shingles" resemble the overlapping scales of a fish and guard the cortex. This thin, colorless layer gives hair its gloss and shine.

*The cortex* is the middle layer. It's here where we find protein chains that make up the hair structure, which determines hair behavior. The cortex is made up of a soft protein, which gives hair its elasticity—its ability to bend and stretch. The softer the protein, the easier it is to style and manipulate the hair. The cortex also contains melanin, the pigment that colors hair. It is also the layer where chemical changes take place when the hair is colored, permed, or relaxed.

*The medulla* is the core of the hair shaft—but not everyone's hair has a medulla. Thick or textured hair usually contains a medulla, while fine and blond hair usually lack this layer. It is made up of large, round, loosely connected cells that contain a protein called keratin. Experts have yet to determine the medulla's true purpose.

## It's All in the Genes!

Your child didn't happen upon her hair by accident; it's hereditary. Hair's texture—how curly or straight it is—is passed along in the family genes, just like eye color. Even if you have stick-straight hair and your child has tight ringlets, that hair type was carried on a chromosome somewhere in her family tree. Genes also determine hair color and when (or if) it will turn gray. Melanin is the pigment made in the skin that gives hair and skin their color. There are two types of melanin: eumelanin (which produces black and brown skin and hair pigment) and phaeomelanin (which produces red and blond skin and hair pigmentation). The ratio of these two pigments gives hair its color:

Blonde: almost no eumelanin and lots of phaeomelanin

Brunette: lots of eumelanin and little phaeomelanin

Red: little eumelanin and lots of phaeomelanin

Dark brown or black: lots of eumelanin and almost no phaeomelanin

## A Few Fascinating Hair Facts

- Hair is almost entirely made of protein: 91 percent.

- Although your body can have more than a million hair follicles growing on it, only 10 percent of that hair is on your head!

- Not everyone has the same amount of hair on her head, and color plays a part. Blondes have about 140,000; brunettes 100,000; and redheads 85,000.

- Each hair follicle has a small muscle attached. These muscles flex and contract to raise the hair away from the body when you are cold or frightened (to keep skin warm and protected). This is called *piloerection,* but is better known as goose bumps.

- The longer your hair is, the older its ends are.

- Girls' hair grows more slowly than boys'.

## Your Child's "Hair-story"

Babies' hair growth patterns can vary widely. Infants often lose all the hair they're born with during their first six months. Sometimes the hair will grow back immediately, but in a totally new color or texture. In other babies, it will take a while to grow back. As your child grows, her hair will continue to change and get thicker, reaching its fullest when she's in her late teens or early twenties.

Scalp hair follicles produce hair at a rate of about ½ inch to 1 inch a month; that's 5 to 6 inches a year. Hair follicles, over time, cycle on and off. The average hair growth cycle lasts between two and seven years and consists of three phases: the *anagen,* the *catagen,* and the *telogen.* In the first phase, the anagen, new cells form in the hair bulb. Eighty to ninety percent of all hair on your head is in this phase at any moment, with every hair at a slightly different stage of the process. The catagen is the next phase, when hair stops growing because cell division stops in the bulb. In the third phase, the telogen, a new hair starts growing from the same follicle and pushes the old hair until it falls out. Most people lose one hundred to two hundred head hairs per day.

The maximum length to which your child can grow her hair is also a matter of genetics. Long hair takes a very long growing cycle to achieve—as much as several years. Some girls can grow Rapunzel-like locks, while others find that getting their hair past their shoulders is impossible because they have shorter growth cycles.

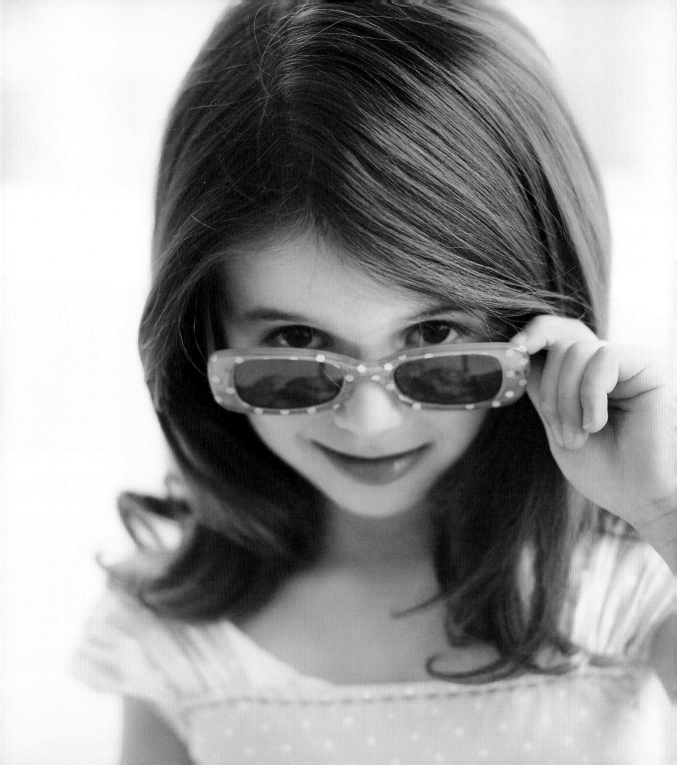

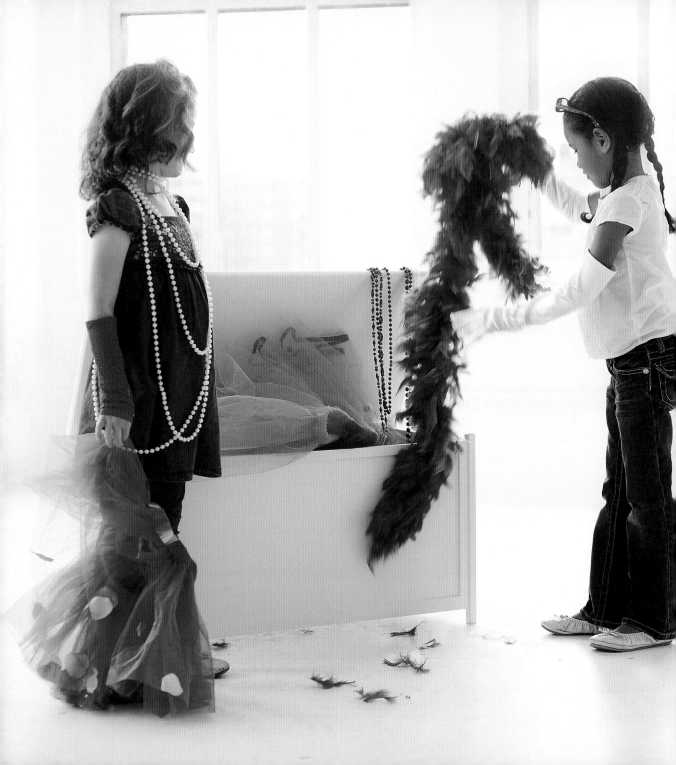

# CHAPTER 2

# *What's Her Type?*

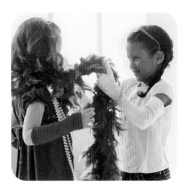

*You think you* know your child, right? She hates broccoli and loves ballet . . . or she's a soccer champ who can't say no to chocolate chip cookies. But how well do you know her hair? Is it curly or wavy? Is it thick or medium? Is it oily or dry or somewhere in between? Hair type can be determined by evaluating three different facets: texture, volume, and condition. Determine where your child falls in each of these categories—combined with her hair length—and you'll know precisely what products and styles will work best for her.

With each of the hairstyles in this book, you'll see the following key that uses symbols to represent hair length (short, medium, or long) and texture (straight, wavy, or curly). Look for the bold white circles to indicate what hair types the style is best suited for. Once you identify your child's hair, you'll be able to refer to this key to see which styles in the book are best for her.

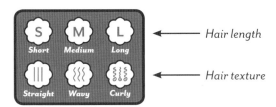

← —— *Hair length*

← —— *Hair texture*

## Straight, Curly, and Wavy

Ever wonder what makes some hair straight and other hair curly? It's complicated, and even researchers can't agree on one theory. Some say it depends on the shape and opening of the hair follicle. If you have curly hair, your follicle probably looks like a squashed circle. Wavy-haired people have oval follicles, and straight-haired people have circular follicles. Other experts say texture is based on the position of the hair bulb inside the follicle. Girls with curls may have a curved end to the hair shaft, making their hair grow at an angle, while straight hair comes from a straight shaft. Finally, some hair experts theorize that chemical bonds that occur between hair proteins are the cause of curliness. The more bonds that naturally occur, the curlier the hair (and vice versa). You'll find a whole chapter in this book (see pages 97–117) dedicated to the special care of straight and curly hair, but here are some basics to get you started.

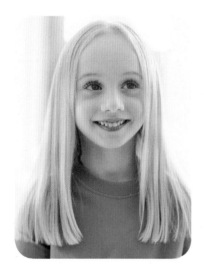

*Straight hair*

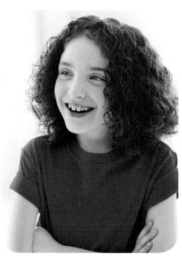

*Curly hair*

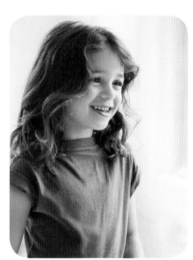

*Wavy hair*

*Straight Hair* You (and your daughter) will love the fact that straight hair rarely tangles and tends to look shinier than curly hair. The only downside to having pin-straight locks is that styling it as anything other than straight can be a challenge; you'll need products, tools, and patience to give very straight hair texture and bend.

**How to handle it:**

- Shampooing with a volumizing product (see page 54) can add lift to limp locks.

- Styling products—like gel, mousse, or hair spray—will help seal and support a style. Though it's tempting to use a curling iron or a blow-dryer to build body, try not to abuse these tools. They'll damage hair, and split ends show easily on straight strands.

- Layered or feathery cuts can give straight hair the appearance of more volume.

*Curly Hair* Curly girls are lucky to have bouncy, fun, springy hair that never lacks volume. Curls come in all shapes and sizes, ranging from loose ringlets to zigzags and tight coils. Curly hair can be either thick or fine. Either way, you'll need to use products that both moisturize and define curls, because humidity in the air stretches them out, making the curls lose their shape and frizz up fast.

**How to handle it:**

- Washing every day can strip the hair of its natural oils, which help keep curls healthy. Instead, aim to shampoo three times a week, and use a curl-enhancing shampoo and conditioner with moisturizers and frizz reducers.

- Look for brands made specially for curly hair. There's a bit of a controversy over whether to brush or comb curly hair after washing. While most stylists agree that brushing is not recommended, many stylists do recommend combing with a wide-tooth comb when hair is wet, especially if your child has thick, hard-to-manage curls. After combing, you may also need to coax them into shape with your fingers.

- Find a stylist who knows how to cut curls (not everyone does) and will work to give the hair a soft, natural shape, rather than an overall pouf.

*Wavy Hair* This is the best of both worlds! It's somewhere between straight and curly hair, so it has a soft, natural bend that you can minimize or maximize, depending on the style you have in mind. Not all wavy hair is the same; it can be fine and thin, medium, or thick and textured. So when you choose shampoos and other products, look for those that cater to the volume of your child's hair. If it's fine, you'll want lightweight products that won't weigh down the wave. And like curly hair, wavy hair can frizz easily and will probably need some coaxing with products and tools to keep its curves.

### How to handle it:

- Shine-enhancing shampoos and conditioners can help this hair type. They maintain its moisture, adding softness and shine without weighing it down.

- To avoid the frizz factor when air-drying wavy hair, blot it dry with a thin smooth towel. You'll achieve a naturally tousled bedhead look.

- Use a wide-tooth comb to detangle wavy hair. Avoid overbrushing (it will just make hair frizzy); instead, scrunch hair with gel or styling cream to shape and smooth.

- The length is key: cut hair too short, and it loses its wave (and gains frizz); grow it too long, and hair is weighed down too much to wave. Somewhere in the middle, with layers, is ideal.

## *Special Hair Types: African American and Asian*

All hair is made up of protein. So what makes some hair look or behave differently? The shape of its follicle and its internal structure play a big part in making hair types unique.

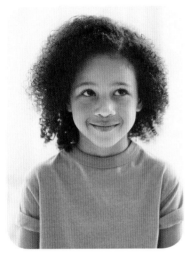

African American hair

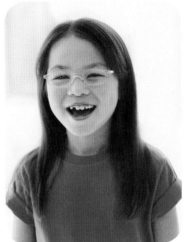

Asian hair

**African American Hair** Tending to be more cortex than cuticle, African American hair has a lot of soft protein, which allows the hair to bend and style easily. This type of hair can be prone to damage, making care and maintenance difficult if you don't understand the techniques. That said, there are so many creative possibilities for styling! Twists, coils, braids . . . the sky's the limit! With a little TLC, this type of hair will look beautiful every day.

**How to handle it:**
- Moisture-rich products, specially formulated for African American hair, make hair easier to shape and style. A deep conditioner once a month is great for maintaining moisture.

- Hair should be shampooed no more than two times per week. Shampooing often removes natural oils from the scalp, which help provide the moisture needed to maintain shine and elasticity. Use a moisture-based shampoo and be as gentle as possible—hair is at its weakest when it is wet.

- When drying, blot the hair rather than rubbing it with the towel. Rubbing will scratch and break the cuticle layers, causing damage. Use a wide-tooth comb and comb out from the ends first. Never use a brush to style; it will make hair frizzy.

- Always use hydrating styling products and leave-in conditioners before blow-drying or using any other heated tool. These products coat and protect the hair.

- When pulling hair back for styles such as ponytails and braids, never pull the hair too tight—it can cause breakage at the hairline.

- Relaxers are not generally recommended for straightening children's hair because they're harsh on the scalp (most experts suggest waiting until your child is a teen to try them). But if you do want to use one, use the gentlest one you can find, and have a professional apply it. Some people instead use a detangling cream with a flat iron to straighten the hair (see page 30). It works—and is less stressful on delicate hair—but the results don't last as long.

- As with all hair types, it is important to find a stylist experienced with your particular needs. Be sure to choose one who specializes in African American hair.

***Asian Hair*** With more layers (close to ten) of cuticle than Caucasian hair (which has about five), Asian hair tends to be straight and heavy, and the scales of the cuticle are wider, thicker, and more densely packed. That's what gives these locks a gorgeous gloss and keeps them strong! Styling this hair type, however, can be trying.

### How to handle it:

- This hair type typically needs moisture products to soften the hard protein in the cuticle layers and allow for more pliability and elasticity.

- Asian hair should be shampooed every other day, because products and everyday dirt and debris build up easily on the heavy cuticle.

- Asian hair tends to resist bending and stretching, so if you want some wave, you'll need the help of a styling tool (such as a curling iron or hot rollers) that will help set the style. Again, go lightly. Don't use heated styling aids more than once a week, or hair will become damaged.

- When using barrettes, look for ones with traction (those with rubber barrette liners or teeth) or French clips that fasten securely. Because of Asian hair's silky texture, regular barrettes tend to slip right out of the hair.

- Asian hair tends to lie very flat. Back-combing can provide volume at the crown or even at the sides when pulling hair back. Also known as *teasing* or *ratting,* this means repeatedly combing the hair toward the scalp, causing the hair to tangle and knot up, which gives it tremendous volume. Or, to avoid actually creating tangles, try a little volumizing cream at the roots.

## Hair Volume

The simplest way to determine the volume of your child's hair is to pull it back into a ponytail. If the base of the ponytail is very slim—about the diameter of a dime—her hair is fine. If the diameter is larger than a quarter, her hair is thick. Another clue: Can you see her scalp when her hair is wet? If so, her hair is probably fine. If you can't see any scalp peeking through, it's thick. If your child's hair falls between these extremes, she probably has medium-volume hair, the most common type.

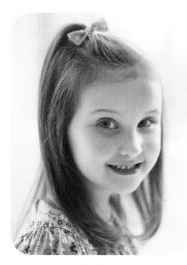

Fine hair

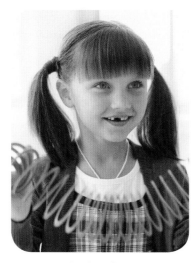

Medium hair

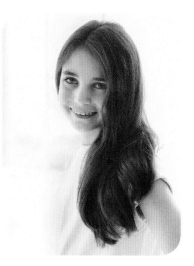

Thick hair

**Fine hair** tends to have more cuticle. That harder protein makes hair shiny and sleek, but also more difficult to style. Warning: Parents tend to overuse products on this type of hair to get it to cooperate. The result is limp hair that's weighed down with product.

**How to handle it:**

- It's important to use a gentle shampoo and a lightweight conditioner (usually just on the ends) on fine hair. Always make sure, when shampooing, to scrub the scalp well with the pads of your fingers (the scalp is where oils come from that tend to make fine hair look oily quickly). This hair type may need shampooing more often, but play around with when to condition (every other day or even once a week may suffice, to avoid weighing it down).

- Stick to liquid-based products (styling sprays) rather than oil- or cream-based ones (styling creams). Spray on roots before blow-drying and blow-dry upside down to add body. And don't be afraid to use a little hair spray if needed.

- The best cuts for fine hair are short, blunt styles that give the illusion of more hair.

*Medium-volume hair* is what most people have. The perfect blend of fine and thick, it has lots of body and usually holds a style well. It's softer and more flexible than thick hair but more voluminous and manageable than fine hair.

**How to handle it:**

- Medium hair can be shampooed and conditioned regularly and styled with multiple products.

- It will generally hold curls fairly easily. Just coat the hair with a protective barrier such as a styling product when using hot tools—either a cream for heavier control or a lightweight liquid product for light protection and softer hold.

- Once a month, apply a deep conditioner to keep hair healthy.

- This type of hair is versatile with most cuts.

*Thick hair* is very strong and has a lot of volume! It looks like there is a lot of hair, and there is: about 150,000 strands, compared to thin-haired types, who have about 90,000 strands. Because there's so much of it, parents often find this hair type a little tough to manage. It can also overwhelm a child's face, especially if it's wavy or curly. So in general, don't be afraid to use products and tools to help tame it.

**How to handle it:**

- Thick hair needs a moisture-based shampoo and conditioner. The weight of these products helps hair lay down and stay calm. Shampoo every other day and use a conditioner each time. Natural oils from the scalp keep hair moisturized, but when hair is thicker, it takes longer for the natural oils to work through—hence the benefit of frequent conditioning.

- Deep-condition hair once or twice a month.

- Oil-based products like shine serum and spray shines are good in moderation for thick hair. They keep it from being frizzy or flyaway.

- Blow-dry with the dryer nozzle facing down to close the cuticle. This will help smooth out the frizzies.

- Regular cuts (every 4 to 6 weeks) are crucial. This will help thin out the hair and maintain its shape.

## Hair Condition

What makes hair dry or oily or somewhere in between? Glands called sebum surround each hair follicle and excrete an oily substance onto the scalp. This oil keeps hair soft and moisturized, but it also attracts dirt. A certain amount of this oil is essential to maintain a healthy scalp, but sometimes the sebum overdo it, and the result is oily hair. When the sebum don't produce enough oil, hair is dry. The right shampoos and conditioners can help. But condition is about more than just natural oil: sun, salt, chlorine, and overstyling can also make strands parched. For more on the effects of environment on hair, see pages 60–61. For information on combating split ends, see page 67.

**Oily hair** looks slightly dull and dirty, especially at the scalp. Strands feel slippery when you run your fingers over them, and tend to look a little limp and stringy.

**How to handle it:** Shampoo more often, at least every other day, with a gentle shampoo, and focus on massaging the shampoo into the scalp.

**Dry hair** looks fuzzy, frizzy, or flyaway, almost like straw. If the scalp is also dry, your child may have dandruff flakes (see page 66).

**How to handle it:** Shampoo only two times a week with a moisturizing shampoo, and always condition—even if you're just giving hair a rinse. If the hair is superdry, you can use a leave-in conditioner as well. Avoid products that contain alcohol, since this can dry hair out even more.

**Combination Hair** As the day goes on, your child's hair starts to look oily around the roots, but the ends remain dry.

**How to handle it:** Shampoo every other day with a shampoo for normal hair and concentrate on the scalp. Use a conditioner, but only on the ends.

**Normal Hair** With hair that is neither oily nor dry, your child has lucked out! You'll just want to keep her hair clean, conditioned, and protected.

**How to handle it:** Shampoo two to three times a week with a gentle shampoo. Follow with conditioner on the ends and a spray-in detangler.

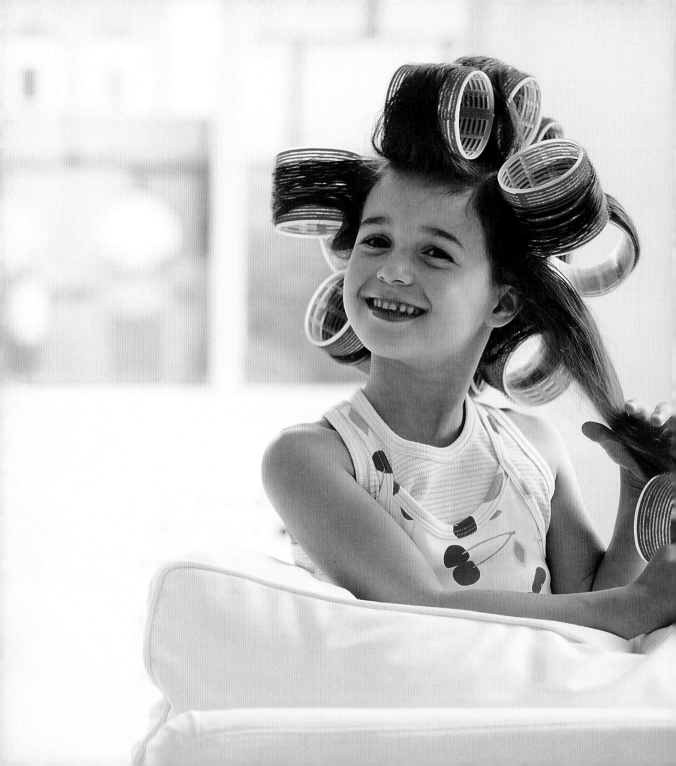

CHAPTER 3

# *Tool School*

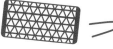

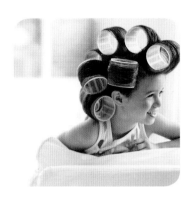

***Browse the shelves*** of any beauty supply shop or drugstore and you'll find dozens of different brushes, combs, blow-dryers, and irons. What should you buy? What do you need? Anything? Everything? Before you go crazy stocking your cart, remember that less is more. Kids will be kids, and their hair should never be too polished. Too much styling will pull out or damage their hair, and fancy styling won't last anyway. Also, blow-drying and curling or straightening are best done only once in a while on kids—no more than once a week—because heat damages the hair so readily. Air-drying (except in cold weather) is much healthier for the hair, and a little detangler and a headband is much faster for parents day to day.

That said, you'll want a few basics in your belt. Each style in this book includes a "What You'll Need" section, which will tell you what tools and accessories are required. Here's a quick course on what each tool does and some tips on what to look for when buying.

## Dryers, Blow by Blow

Ever wonder how a blow-dryer works? The basic version consists simply of a metal coil that heats up in the dryer when an electrical current passes through it. An electric motor blows the hot air out through a nozzle. While these dryers serve their purpose—they literally blow the water out of your hair—they also dry out the hair itself, making it look frizzy and flyaway. Luckily, there are many better options.

**Ionic Hair Dryers** Any heating element, whether on an electric stove or in a hair dryer, produces positively charged particles called positive ions. Positive ions from a hair dryer cause the cuticle of the hair shaft to open, which lets essential moisture evaporate. The result: hair can easily become dehydrated. Negative ions, however, do the reverse: They seal the cuticle of each hair shaft, keeping moisture in. Ionic dryers produce only negative ions, which attach to positive ions in the hair, making it shiny, smooth, and static free. An ionic dryer also dries your hair up to 50 percent faster than regular dryers; less prolonged heat on the hair means less damage.

**Ceramic Hair Dryers** Ceramic dryers have a heating coil that is made of ceramic rather than metal. Ceramic is a superconductor—unlike metal, it heats evenly, which means it isn't likely to become hot enough to damage hair. Ceramic dryers also produce negative ions—so they offer a double advantage! If your child's hair tends to be frizzy or unmanageable, ceramic or tourmaline dryers (see below) are your best bet. They help straighten hair and make it smooth and shiny. You'll find that these dryers are more expensive, but they're usually worth the price: They're better for the hair's health and better for styling. They also won't spark or short out, so they will last longer than traditional dryers.

**Tourmaline Hair Dryers** These hair dryers are considered the ultimate in hair drying. They have industrial-grade tourmaline (pronounced TUR-muh-leen) gemstones in their coils, which are claimed to produce even more negative ions, up to six times more than ceramic. You may find ionic and ceramic dryers that also have tourmaline components. These dryers can be very pricey—costing as much as $300—but you can find models for as little as $30 that get good reviews from *Good Housekeeping, Consumer Reports,* and others.

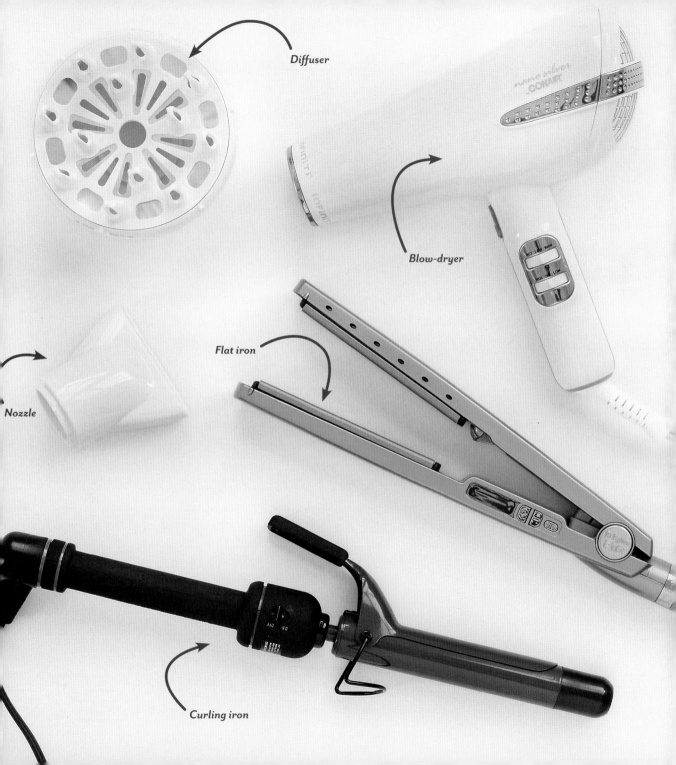

Diffuser

Blow-dryer

Nozzle

Flat iron

Curling iron

Once you have chosen a type of hair dryer, there are a few other features to consider. Dryers with different speed and heat levels are best for kids with fine or delicate hair, because they put you in control. The higher the wattage of your hair dryer, the more powerful the speed and heat will be. The recommended average wattage for a dryer is 1,750 watts, and this is plenty for a child's hair. You can protect hair from damage simply by turning the speed and heat down. Generally, you should use the higher speed and heat settings to remove excess water when you begin drying, then switch to lower settings for more precise styling. If hair is very dry or damaged, use the lowest setting the entire time.

If styling your child's hair is difficult (it simply won't hold a curl or flip), then having a cool-shot button on your dryer can make a big difference. Heated hair is more pliable and can easily lose its shape. But cooling the hair quickly (for about 5 seconds) with a blast of cool air as you hold the style can lock it in.

There are also various attachments for dryers. If hair is curly or wavy, a diffuser is helpful. A diffuser diffuses, or spreads, the air coming out of the dryer, so it doesn't come out in one hot blast. Some diffusers even come with prongs on the end so curls can be lifted as they're dried. A conelike nozzle attachment is a plus for straightening any kind of hair; it focuses the air directly where you need it.

Finally, there are practical considerations. Lightweight or compact dryers may be easier for you to handle (not to mention travel with), especially when you're trying to use a brush or keep a squirming child still while you style. If your child has very long hair that takes more than ten minutes to dry, you'll probably want to purchase a lighter model (weighing 2 to 3 pounds or less) to prevent your arms from aching. Retractable cords are a plus around young children, who might be tempted to play with the cord. Some dryers come with a wall mount, which is helpful for keeping them out of small hands. There are also low-noise dryers, which are great for young children who might be frightened of the roar of a regular dryer.

## Info on Irons

**Curling Irons** Most girls with straight hair dream of having a head full of curlicues (we all want what we don't have, right?). The right curling iron can grant that wish. Curling irons can create soft waves, bouncy ringlets, or tight coils, depending on what type and size you use. As with hair dryers, materials make a difference. Most irons are made of metal and coated in gold, titanium, ceramic, or tourmaline. Ceramic and tourmaline are considered top-of-the-line. Ceramic ionic technology eliminates frizz in the same way a hair dryer does by providing even heat distribution, and tourmaline infused into the plates delivers negative ions to make hair extra smooth and shiny. A steam curling iron (one that you add water to) is good for hard-to-curl hair; the steam locks the curls into place. Steam is also less damaging than dry heat—a plus for delicate hair.

Different curling irons will provide different types of curls; the bigger the barrel of the iron, the looser the curl. So a ¾-inch curling iron will create tight spirals while a 2-inch one will make softer waves. The length and thickness of your child's hair should also be a consideration when choosing the barrel diameter. For short or fine hair, a barrel size of ¾ to 1¼ inches is ideal; for medium-length and medium-thickness hair, go with a 1- to 1½-inch barrel; for long (below the shoulder) or thick hair, a 1¼- to 2½-inch curling iron is recommended. A cordless version is handy for traveling and also easier to handle; there are no wires to get in the way.

## Dear Cozy,

*My curling iron seems to have so many temperature settings on it. What temp is best to use on my child's hair?*

*As a guideline, if your child has fine/thin hair, set the iron to below 180 degrees (low); for normal hair, 180–190 degrees (medium); for textured or thick hair, 190–210 degrees (high). Do not leave hair wrapped around the barrel for more than a few seconds. Any longer and you'll scorch the strands.*

***Flat Irons*** Also known as straightening irons, flat irons also vary in size, technology, and price. You may want to use one *occasionally* on your child if her hair is curly, wavy, frizzy, or hard to manage. A flat iron is simple to use—just clamp a small section of hair a few inches from the scalp (so as not not to burn it) between the two plates and gently pull down to the ends. Hair is instantly straighter, smoother, and shinier.

The technology includes the same ionic, ceramic, and tourmaline options as those for curling irons (see page 29). Prices on these irons can range from $20 to $300 for the top-of-the-line tourmaline models, but a decent flat iron should cost you about $50. Be sure when you buy a ceramic or tourmaline iron that it is truly made of these materials, not just coated with them. It will say so on the box. Also, look for the words "PTC heater" on the box (PTC stands for positive temperature coefficient); most of the better models will have it. This type of heating element radiates slow, even heat that protects hair strands and helps seal in moisture.

Straightening irons, like curling irons, come in different sizes. The longer and thicker your child's hair, the bigger the iron surface you want. A 1-inch iron is recommended for thin to medium thickness and short to medium lengths; 2-inch models are best suited for girls with long, thick, or curly hair. Also, longer plates make straightening easier; look for plates that span the length of the entire clamp. An iron with variable heat settings will allow you more control and you can use it on different hair types in your family; fine hair needs less heat to style, while thick hair needs more. Some irons have interchangeable styling plates for straightening or crimping, allowing you more styling options—and it's always a good idea to look for a model with an automatic safety shutoff.

## Heat Helpers

Heating tools can crack and damage the hair cuticle. There are many products that buffer heat from flat irons, curling irons, blow-dryers, and rollers while enhancing the effectiveness of each appliance. Spray, serum, lotion, gel? All of them promise to protect your child's hair, and technically all of them will, just by adding a layer of coating between her hair and the superhot temperature of your tool. For kids, look for a heat protectant that's lightweight to the touch, heat-activated, and packed with healthy ingredients (such as vitamin E or amino acids).

## Let's Roll!

Rollers—both heated and unheated—are another great way to give hair some wave, curl, or body. They vary in length and width; a wide diameter gives a full, soft curl, while a thin roller gives a tight spiral. You can have fun experimenting with different sizes and how many you use—just a few at the hairline or a whole head of bouncy ringlets.

Magnetic rollers are hard plastic cylinders with ventilation holes—the traditional kind you might see in old-fashioned beauty parlors. They're not really magnetic; they get their name from the fact that hair seems to stick to them. Hair needs to be wet when using this type of roller—so the curling process will take as long as it takes for hair to completely dry (which is why women often sit under a hooded dryer at the salon). They're rigid rollers, so not supercomfy for a kid's head, but if your child has hard-to-curl hair, these will usually do the trick. You can run a blow-dryer over the set to help the drying along.

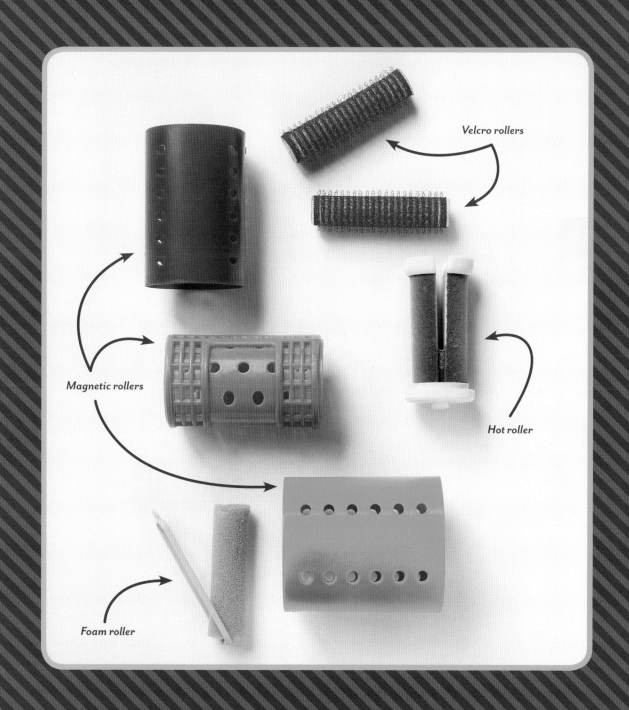

Velcro rollers

Magnetic rollers

Hot roller

Foam roller

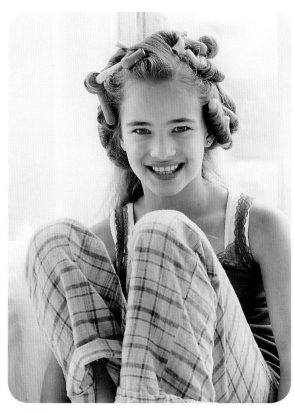

*Foam rollers* are supersoft and gentle, and can give curl to fragile hair. They are best used on dry hair, and are even soft enough to sleep on, for lasting results.

*Velcro rollers* provide soft curl and can be used on either damp or dry hair. Just roll in the direction you want the wave or curl; the Velcro "sticks" to the hair and unrolls gently and easily with no tugging. The length of time needed to leave the rollers in depends on your hair type. For straighter hair, leaving the rollers in longer will provide a better curl that will last longer. If putting rollers in wet hair, using a blow-dryer will help lock in curls. If your child's hair is long or thick, you might need to use pinch clips or bobby pins to keep Velcro rollers in place.

*Hot rollers and steam rollers* are great when you need a do *fast*. Plug in the set, wait for the rollers to heat up, and then roll the hair. Both types are used on dry hair to create long-lasting curl and minimize frizz (some high-end sets are even ionic, so they boost shine), and they're less damaging to hair than curling irons. Just be careful not to leave heated rollers in a child's hair too long: Remove them when they're cool enough to touch (just a few minutes after putting them in the hair) because once they cool they can be tough to unroll. The dry heat can also damage the hair, which is why a steam roller set may be more desirable, especially for fine or delicate hair.

## Comb and Brush Basics

Depending on your child's hair and the styles you want to achieve, you may want to have a few combs and brushes handy. Combs are often used first, to detangle and part the hair; then a brush is used for drying and styling.

You should clean combs and brushes regularly—at least once a month—so as not to add dirt and buildup to the hair while styling it. Remove any hair from the comb or brush, then rinse with warm water and a mild soap or shampoo. It's also a good idea to replace brushes once a year, especially if some bristles have come out or become broken. They can scratch a child's delicate scalp.

### Combs

A wide-tooth comb is ideal for detangling. Because the teeth are so far apart, they are less likely to pull hair; look for one with rounded tips on the teeth, which will be gentle on the scalp. Use a wide-tooth comb on wet strands straight out of the shower/bath/pool or to evenly distribute styling product such as gel or mousse through hair. A fine-tooth comb will help you part hair or create sections for complicated dos.

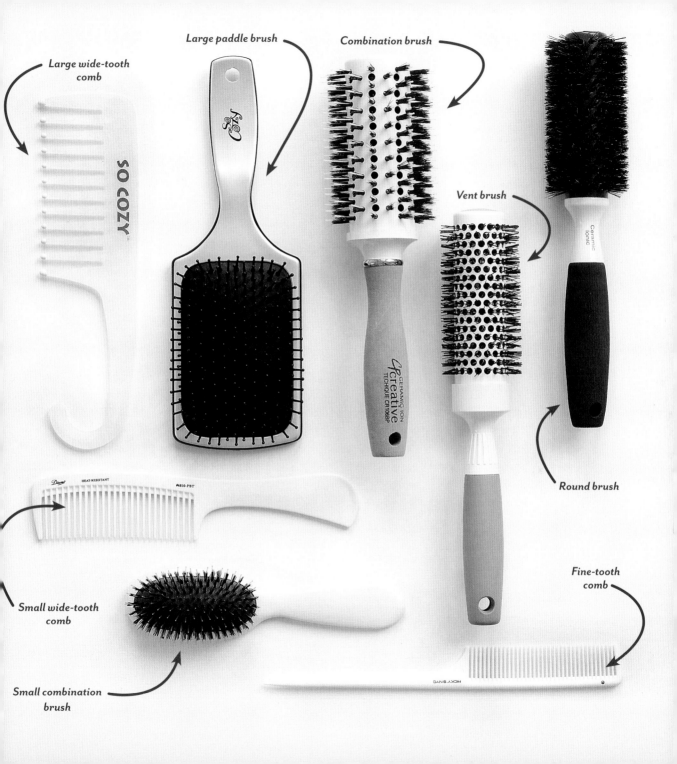

*Large wide-tooth comb*

*Large paddle brush*

*Combination brush*

*Vent brush*

*Round brush*

*Small wide-tooth comb*

*Small combination brush*

*Fine-tooth comb*

## Brushes

There are two things to consider when choosing a brush: shape and bristle material. Choose the shape based on your child's hair type and how you tend to style it, then consider bristle material.

**Round brushes** give a lift and a slight bend to the hair when used for styling. Choose a brush with a small diameter if hair is fine or layered; a large diameter works best for thicker and longer hair. And they're great for blowouts (see page 116) because they grip the hair firmly.

**Paddle brushes** are flat and wide. They're ideal for smoothing and straightening most types of long hair. These brushes perform better than a round brush for basic brushing of dry hair because there is less danger of tangling.

**Vent brushes** allow hair to dry quickly because of vents in the base of the brush beneath the bristles. Using a vent brush for blow-drying allows warm air to circulate and decreases drying time—and less drying time means less danger of damage to the hair.

As for bristles, nylon bristle brushes are affordable and allow hair to slide through the bristles without any pulling or snagging. The only negative: Nylon bristles have a tendency to create static electricity. Boar bristle brushes are made of actual boar hair, which is similar to human hair in structure. They are gentle on the hair and scalp and have natural antistatic properties. Boar bristles are recommended for fine or medium-volume hair—the bristles are too soft for thick hair.

You can also try a combination bristle brush, which has both boar and nylon bristles. The nylon bristles among the boar bristles help the brush penetrate the hair while still being gentle on the scalp. Boar or combination brushes may be a little more expensive, but they are better for the hair and will probably also last longer than cheap plastic or synthetic bristle brushes, which can scratch the scalp or even melt under dryer heat.

## Eating for Healthy Hair

It's not just what you use on your child's head—it's what goes into her body as well. Nutritionists say it's a good idea to encourage your child to eat a variety of these healthy foods.

- Peanuts, corn, and spinach contain vitamin E, which stimulates hair growth.

- Folic acid, found in foods like asparagus, peas, citrus fruits, and turkey, will help promote long locks by strengthening strands so they don't break.

- Vitamin B produces keratin, a protein that strengthens strands. Eat bananas, whole-grain cereals, rice, and eggs.

- Dairy products like skim milk and yogurt—as well as broccoli and strawberries—are great sources of calcium, an important mineral for hair growth.

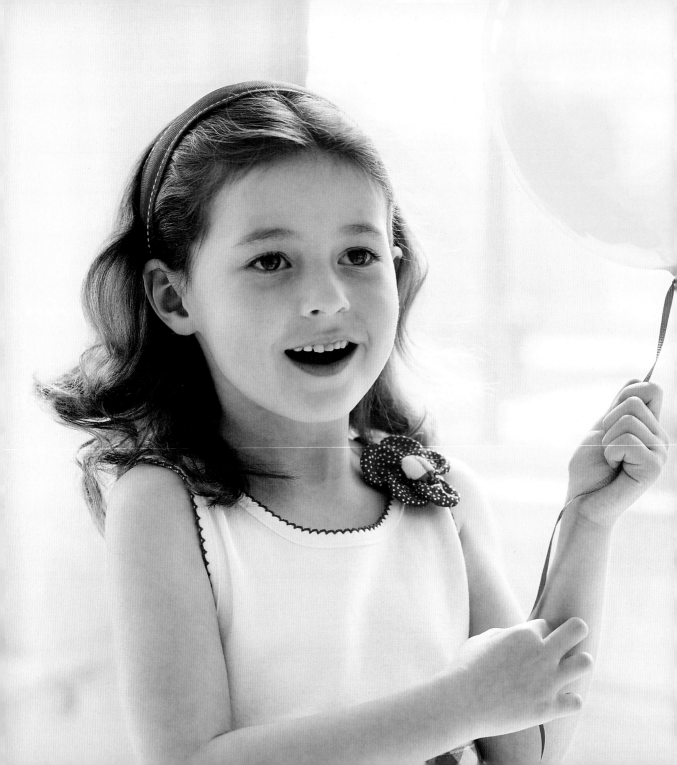

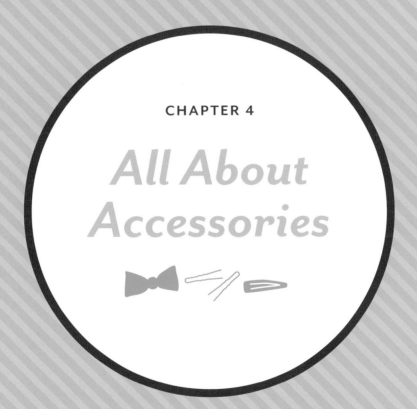

CHAPTER 4

*All About
Accessories*

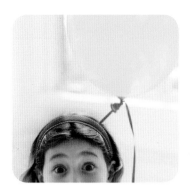

*The perfect barrette,* headband, or ponytail holder is a little special touch, like jewelry for the hair—but accessories can also be the perfect tools for creating fast, no-fuss styles for everyday wear. After all, what is simpler than a ponytail?

Most girls love to collect hair accessories. You can start small with a few clips for a baby or toddler, then build to a whole box or drawer filled with options for a teen. Let them choose a few styles and colors or even make their own (see page 46)—it's an easy way to unleash creativity and individuality.

## Ponytail Holders

Also known as pony-o's, elastics, or hair ties, these stretchy, elasticized bands can be used to create hundreds of different styles, from classic ponytails to intricate braids and elegant updos. Ouchless or snag-free ponytail holders are covered with a snag-free material that glides against hair rather than gripping it, as rubber does. As the name implies, these pull the hair less, so do less damage. Regular rubber bands should never be used—only those made for hair. In general, a standard medium-sized ponytail holder (about 2 inches in diameter) works for most hair types. For small braids or fine hair, mini-elastics (about ¼ to ¾ of an inch in diameter) are needed. And if you have thick hair, large or oversized holders will work well. The simplest ponytail holders are plain or colored Os that can be bought in bulk, but fancy ones are available with everything from decorative disks to fur pompoms to dangling beads attached. If an elastic ever gets caught in the hair, don't yank! Use a small scissors to snip it out.

**Scrunchies**   And you thought these went out with the 1980s? Kids love them! These elastic bands are encased in a strip of soft fabric that ruffles or bunches up around the band. They come in pretty patterns, colors, and styles (some even have studs or hanging ribbons). Use one to make a quick bun or ponytail. The style will be loose and a little messy . . . but that's the look.

## Hair Clips

This is a generic term for a wide variety of hair accessories. Hair clips pull hair back away from the face by clamping or snapping down on a section of hair. They range from simple to elaborate and come in all sizes. In general, the finer the hair, the smaller the clip should be—and vice versa for longer, thicker strands.

**Barrettes** Although the majority of barrettes are metal, they can be made from a wide variety of materials, from plastic to wood, and decorated with anything from beads to "gems" to bows. Available in small, medium, and large sizes, barrettes snap or clasp closed to hold a portion of hair in place.

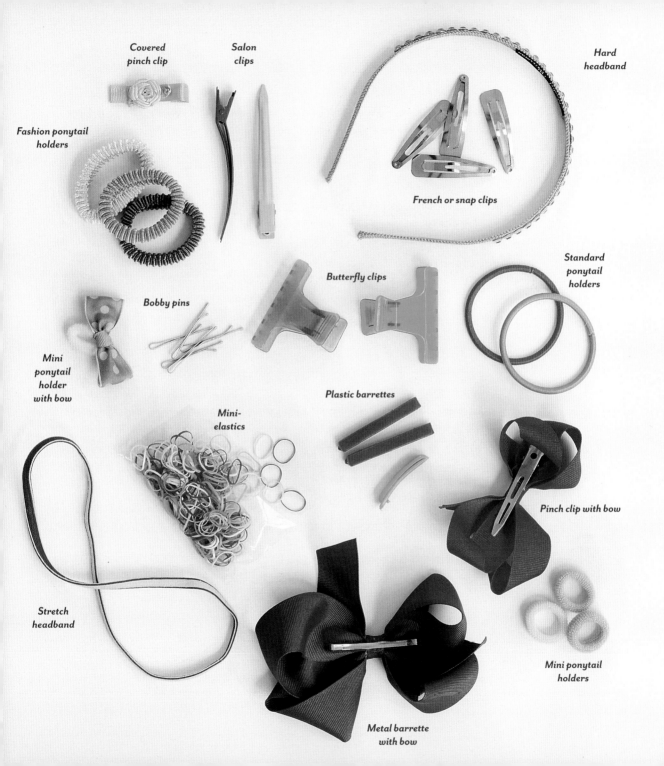

Covered pinch clip

Salon clips

Hard headband

Fashion ponytail holders

French or snap clips

Standard ponytail holders

Butterfly clips

Bobby pins

Mini ponytail holder with bow

Plastic barrettes

Mini-elastics

Pinch clip with bow

Stretch headband

Mini ponytail holders

Metal barrette with bow

**Butterfly Clips** Also called claw or jaw clips, these come in sizes ranging from small to extra large. You squeeze them open and gather together a portion of hair in the jaw or claw. Larger jaw clips can pull back larger portions of hair and secure a whole twist or ponytail. Mini ones are good for fine hair and adorning minibraids or twists.

**Pinch Clips** Also called salon clips, these pinch on one end to open. Pinch clips are great for toddlers who don't like to wear things in their hair because they are very easy for parents to put in—your child may not even notice it. They're good for fine hair or kids who don't have a lot of hair.

**French Clips or Snap Clips** This clip flexes in the center to open and close.

**Hair Snaps** Used mainly for decorative purposes, hair snaps are tiny clips that hold only a few strands. These are ideal for babies and toddlers or for adorning minibraids or twists. However, because of the small size of these, parents should be careful. Letting a child put a hair snap in her mouth would be a choking hazard.

**Hairpins and bobby pins** slide into the hair rather than clamping down. They are great for securing any little loose strands hanging out of a style or for fastening buns or fancy updos in place. Always keep a pile handy in a plastic bag or box. In general, hairpins (which look like a narrow U) are better with thicker hair and for securing large loops or coils like a chignon or bun; bobby pins (which have no space between the prongs) are better for finer hair because they actually hold it together.

## Headbands and Wraps

Headbands and wraps hold hair back away from the face and are a great way to keep kids' hair out of their eyes for school or sports. Some are made of rigid materials like plastic or metal, with or without gripping combs on the inside rim, and rest on the head behind the ears. Other headbands and wraps are made of soft elastic or stretchy fabric and wrap completely around the head. If your young child complains that a hard band gives her a headache, then a soft one is the way to go—it's both pretty and practical.

## Cool Ways to Keep Clips

Your kid has a ton of hair accessories . . . but how can you keep them neat and organized and not just in a heap? Here are some creative ideas.

- Pick up a bead storage box in a craft store. Have your child adorn it with paint, markers, or stickers. Put barrettes in one section, ponytail holders in another, bows in another. If her collection is too big for one, you can stack several.

- Designate a drawer in the bathroom for hair stuff. Use a kitchen utensil separator (the tray-style kind that holds forks and knives) to organize.

- Fill snack-sized baggies or small clear cosmetic bags with same-type accessories and store in a drawer.

- Hang a pretty ribbon or two from the wall and clip hair doodads onto them.

- A tackle box is large enough to store small accessories as well as a brush, a comb, and even a spray bottle. Again, let your little Picasso decorate it.

- A large fold-out hanging cosmetic bag (the kind you'd pack on a trip) makes a great hair accessory holder. You can hang it on the back of the closet or bathroom door.

- Photo storage boxes or small hat boxes (especially ones in bright, pretty colors or patterns) make great accessory keepers.

- One creative mom fills a lunch box with all her daughter's hair goodies. Inside, she uses snack-sized plastic tubs with lids to sort them.

- Hang small tiered baskets in the bathroom or closet and drop accessories into them.

- Recycle any type of box—such as an old chess box (the kind with drawers beneath that store the pieces)—as a bow keeper.

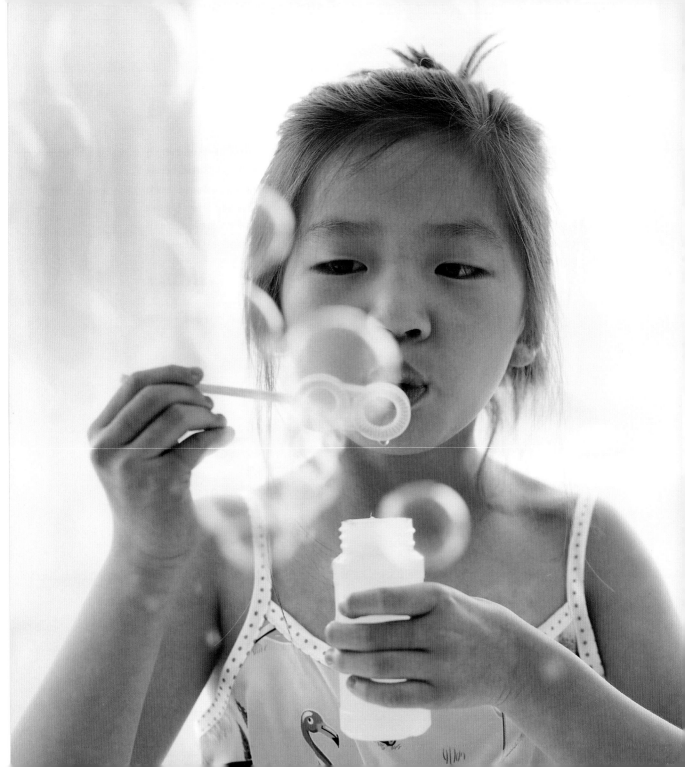

CHAPTER 5

# *Products 101*

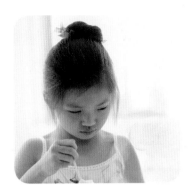

**Why is it** that so many moms with fabulous manes don't have a clue when it comes to their child's hair? It's because a child's hair has different needs than an adult's and requires different products and styling techniques. A child's hair is completely untouched and unaltered; it has never been colored, permed, or processed, and that makes it finer than adult hair and more prone to knotting. So what you'd do for your hair doesn't necessarily go for your daughter's. Kids' hair needs some TLC . . . but that's what parents do best, right?

## Coming Clean About Shampoo

When your child is little, she may hate having her hair washed for any number of reasons: Some kids don't like the water dripping down their face, some are scared of getting shampoo in their eyes, and some just don't want to sit still. There's a lot you can do to make the process less of a chore for both of you. First off, you may want to use a shower attachment to gently sprinkle her hair with water (don't let it run over her face like you would with your own). Also, never underestimate the power of entertainment. Pick up a few tub toys or bright, colorful bottles of shampoo/conditioner and bubble bath to distract her. Sing songs ("I'm singing in the rain! Just singing in the rain!"), make up silly stories, crank up a shower radio. Young children might even like to shampoo their doll while their own hair is being washed.

As your child gets older, washing her hair will get easier; just be sure to choose products that are good for her hair type. For heads of any age, there is a technique to washing: Pour a quarter-sized amount of shampoo into your hand and focus on lathering at the roots—it is the oil-producing scalp that you're washing when you wash hair. Massage the scalp *gently* with your fingertips (not nails) to loosen dirt. Hit the ends last and just work the suds down, don't scrub. There's also no need—unless your kid has super-oily hair—to rinse and repeat. One lather is plenty. Conditioning comes with few rules (see page 56), but remember to focus on the hair strands rather than the scalp in this case—it's the hair that needs the moisture. If your daughter insists on doing it herself, show her how to do it, then check to make sure all the shampoo or conditioner is rinsed out (no soapy suds left behind ears or at the nape of the neck). Read on for the different types of products that are available in formulas for children's hair, and how to use them.

**Tear-free Shampoos** For young kids, it's best to choose a shampoo that's tear-free; that way if suds get into kids' eyes, they won't sting. Adult shampoos typically contain surfactants (the ingredient that creates the suds) and other preservatives that are often irritants that can cause eyes to sting. Children's shampoo formulas typically contain very mild surfactants and counter-irritants that prevent eyes from stinging. These types of shampoos are usually very mild, soap-free, hypoallergenic, and dermatologist-tested. See chapter 2 for more on shampoos and conditioners for different hair types.

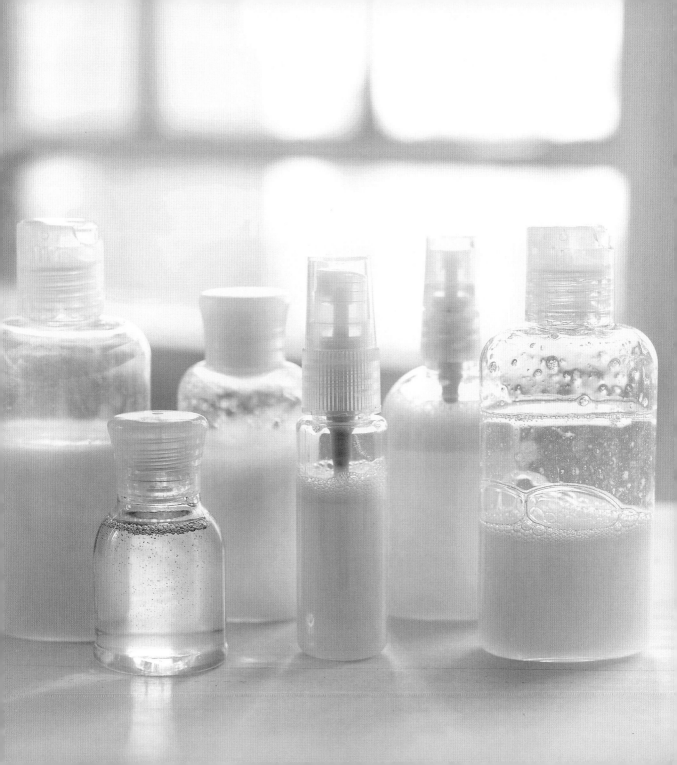

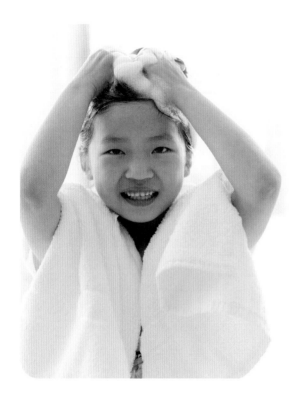

**Clarifying Shampoos** Stuff builds up on your child's hair: dirt, products, hard water and mineral deposits; chlorine and chemicals from swimming pools; even the waxes and moisturizers in some shampoos and conditioners can leave buildup after repeated use. This buildup can cause hair to look dull and feel heavy, greasy, or limp. A clarifying shampoo removes deposits and gives hair a fresh start. It's a good idea to use one once a week if hair is oily (see page 21), once a month if hair is normal or dry.

**Volumizing Shampoos** These shampoos often contain protein (from wheat or rice), which creates a bond with strands of hair, plumping them up by creating a thicker strand. These shampoos can be good for strengthening or building body in fine hair, but these boosting formulas can also build up and eventually weigh hair down—so you don't want to use them every day. Use every few days, switching off with a shampoo that clarifies.

**Hydrating Shampoos** These cleansers contain humectants (such as glycerine), which absorb water from their environment. The shampoo deposits the humectants into the hair, and the humectants help the hair absorb and retain moisture.

### What's in That Shampoo?

Reading a kids' shampoo bottle label is like trying to translate another language! What do all these long chemical-sounding names mean—and what do they do for a child's hair and scalp? Shampoo, by definition, is a liquid formula that contains detergents meant to wash away oil and dirt. But it is important not to strip all the natural oils from the skin and scalp, since these act as a natural barrier to bacteria. Most kids' shampoos are formulated with gentler, tear-free ingredients. As a child grows and becomes more active and exposed to the environment, and her diet changes, she may require a slightly stronger shampoo. Here is a sampling of some common ingredients you'll see on the label of kids' shampoo. All of these ingredients, whether natural or synthetic, are purified and/or processed in commercial chemical manufacturing plants. Like food ingredients, these are listed on the label in order of most to least amount in the product.

- **C:PEG-80 Sorbitan Laurate**—This is a gentle foaming agent that functions as a surfactant ("surface acting agent"). Basically, that means that it serves as a wetting agent, to help reduce surface tension in the water and promote smooth spreading of the shampoo. Surfactants help to remove oil and cleanse the hair. This is a gentler surfactant than the chemicals (such as sodium lauryl sulfate) used in adult shampoos.

- **Sodium Trideceth Sulfate**—Another surfactant, this is a mild cleansing agent with conditioning properties.

- **Citric Acid**—Adjusts the pH of the shampoo to help smooth the hair. A slightly acid pH is desirable so that the hair will be sleek and shiny in appearance—the slight acidity causes the cuticle (or scales on the hair shaft; see page 4) to lie flat, making the hair feel smooth and look shiny. Also, citric acid helps prevent bacterial growth in the shampoo better than other acids.

- **Cocamidopropyl Betaine (CAPB)**—This synthetic surfactant is derived from coconut oil.

- **Hydrolyzed Wheat Protein and Hydrolyzed Wheat Starch**—Combined, these form a hydrating complex that offers moisture-balancing and film-forming properties that work together to give hair better body and a smoother, softer feel.

- Methyl Chloroisothiazolinone, Methyl Isothiazolinone, and Magnesium Chloride—Preservatives with antibacterial and antifungal effects.

- Sodium Hydroxymethylglycinate—A broad-spectrum preservative effective against bacteria, yeast, and mold in the shampoo bottle.

- Tetrasodium EDTA—An agent that neutralizes trace minerals on hair and reduces buildup.

## All About Conditioners

A lot of parents skip this step—mainly because their kids don't want to sit still for any more hair washing. It's very subjective; there is no right or wrong way to use conditioning products. Trial and error is the best way to figure out what's right for your child. Some people like to use a conditioner in the tub daily, whereas others prefer to use a spray-on, leave-in conditioner (it detangles, too). Some like to use both if hair is very dry. Using a styling product that conditions the hair is another way to help keep the hair hydrated and healthy. One helpful rule of thumb is the drier the hair, the more conditioning you need for it to be healthy. And remember, whenever you condition, concentrate on the ends, not the roots, where conditioner can weigh hair down and make it look limp.

**Detangler** This step is even more important than conditioning. Choose a deeply moisturizing leave-in spray; it won't just erase knots, it will also strengthen strands. One trick professional stylists use is to dilute the leave-in detangler with a few drops of water so it doesn't weigh hair down or feel sticky.

## Organic Products

The jury is still out about the importance of natural and organic hair care products and the implications of using artificial or synthetic ingredients. The recent touting of "all natural" ingredients in the industry is based more on marketing trends than on conclusive findings. Artificial preservatives and synthetics aren't all bad. Think of organic food: generally speaking, organic is preferable to nonorganic, but that doesn't mean that all nonorganic food options are bad. Very often your choices are limited. It's similar for organic hair care products. Furthermore, manufacturers have had a difficult time formulating organic styling products that are effective—meaning these formulations often do not prevent frizz, provide hold, or add volume.

Knowing the truth is also difficult. Currently the FDA has very loose regulations regarding the classification and labeling of hair care products. Many claim to be organic when in fact they may have just one organic ingredient. There are very few 100 percent organic products on the market. Some products claim to be all natural when in fact they are loaded with synthetic ingredients. Buyers beware: Read the ingredient list *carefully* if you're trying to choose organic.

## Should I Worry About Parabens?

Parabens are preservatives that are added to beauty products to keep them from growing bacteria and to increase their shelf life. They are widely used in the cosmetic industry and have, until recently, been considered safe. But recent studies have linked parabens to increased estrogen levels and increased risks of cancer in people who have been exposed to them. A study published in 2004 in the *Journal of Applied Toxicology* detected parabens in breast tumors. Additionally, it's thought that babies absorb through their skin almost three times the chemicals in soaps and bath products that adults do. So even though, at this time, the FDA believes "there is no reason for consumers to be concerned," as a parent, you may want to avoid any parabens in your child's hair products.

When you read the label of a hair care product, look for the following ingredients: *methylparaben, proplyparaben, isopropylparaben, isobutylparaben, butylparaben, sodium butylparaben.* Since each ends in the word *paraben,* they're pretty easy to spot. Also, many children's hair products are now labeled "paraben-free" as manufacturers are moving to remove them from their kids' lines.

# Knot Know-How: How to Detangle Hair

*By far, the most frequent question asked about children's hair care is, "How do I comb the knots out of my child's hair?" This ouchless technique will work every time—even on the most matted of manes.*

### What You'll Need

Wide-tooth comb

Hair clip to section the hair

Spray leave-in conditioner or
  detangler

Toy, video, or book
  (to keep your kid occupied!)

**Step 1:** Make sure your child is distracted; this is half the battle! Start by parting the hair horizontally from ear to ear and clipping the upper section of hair onto the top of the head, to keep it out of the way. (For more on how to section hair, see page 59.)

**Step 2:** Spray the lower (unclipped) section with a leave-in conditioner or detangler.

**Step 3:** Once you've sprayed the section, separate a chunk of hair (a 1- to 2-inch section) and hold it firmly with one hand near the hair ends. Most people's instinct is to comb the hair straight down, starting from the roots. This is not only painful, but also compounds the snags and makes them worse (you can even get the comb stuck in the hair!). Instead, start at the ends and work your way up to the scalp, one inch at a time, gently combing through. Holding the hair just above the snag you're working will prevent tugging on the scalp, which is what hurts. As you work your way up, adjust your hold on the hair.

**Step 4:** Once you've finished the entire bottom section, unclip the rest of the hair and work the top section the same way, in small chunks around the head until you're finished.

# How to Section Hair

*Sectioning is very important. The purpose of sectioning hair is to create an organized area to allow you to work methodically around the entire head, creating neat hairstyles. Trying to work on an entire head of hair can seem overwhelming, but by breaking it down into sections, it becomes much more manageable. Keep in mind that these instructions are for basic sectioning; different hair types and hairstyles require different methods of sectioning. If you are sectioning hair to braid or style it, follow the specific sectioning instructions given with that style.*

### What You'll Need
Wide-tooth comb or brush          Hair clips
Fine-tooth comb

**Step 1:** Brush or comb hair so there are no tangles. Using a fine-tooth comb and starting at the crown of the head (the topmost part), make a straight line down the middle of the back of the head. Gather the hair on one side together and clip it out of the way (illus. 1).

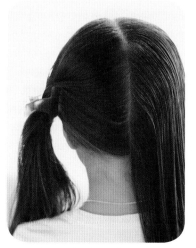
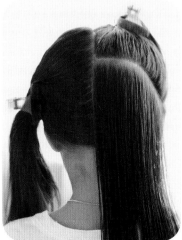
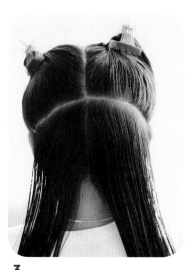

1                              2                              3

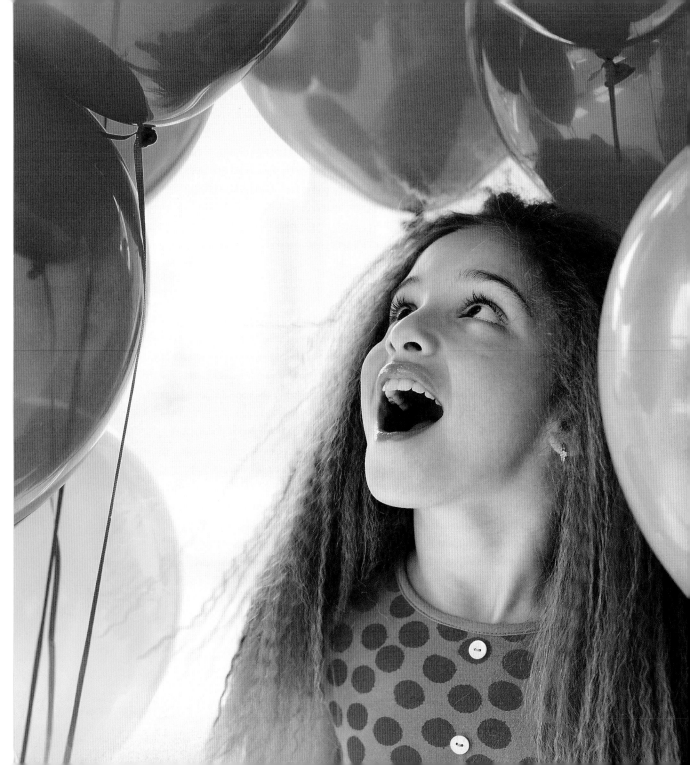

CHAPTER 6

# Hair Emergency!

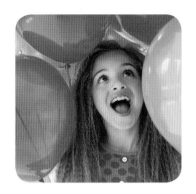

**Your child is** bound to come home one day with a scary, hairy situation. While your first instinct is probably to panic, try to keep your cool around your kid. If you freak, she'll freak—and most of these are not only common problems, but completely fixable. Take a deep breath and read on. . . .

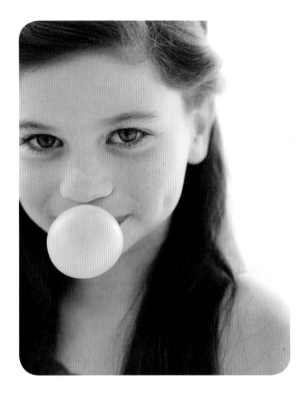

## Gum and Goo

Your kid has a wad of chewing gum (or some other sticky treat) stuck in her hair. Don't go nuts. Instead, cover the area with smooth peanut butter (the oilier the better), and gently glide your fingers down the hair strands, using your thumbnail to dislodge the gum. Be sure to hold the hair above the gum with your free hand to prevent tugging on the scalp. Repeat until the hair is gum-free, then shampoo as normal. All gone!

## Dandruff

You notice (and probably everyone else does, too) snowy white flakes all over your child's shoulders. Dandruff isn't contagious or dangerous, but it can be a bit itchy and embarrassing. Lots of things can cause dandruff. Some doctors think it's caused by a fungus that makes the scalp shed skin cells too quickly. Or your child could be peeling from a sunburn on her scalp, or may be using too much shampoo and not rinsing it out well. Other possibilities include conditions such as eczema and psoriasis, which are hereditary.

Once you've ruled out all of the above with a pediatrician so you know you are just dealing with mild dandruff, there are several things you can do to alleviate the problem. A simple solution to treat dandruff is to shampoo more frequently. Before washing, brush your child's hair from the scalp outward along the hair with steady, firm strokes. This will carry oil from the scalp, where it can cause dandruff, along the hair strands, which need the oil to stay shiny and healthy. If this doesn't do the trick, ask your doctor if you can try a medicated dandruff shampoo (these contain tar or salicylic acid, so make sure the pediatrician says whatever you're using is safe for kids).

## Green Hair

Your kid aced her deepwater swim test this summer, but her hair is paying the price: her once golden blond locks have taken on a ghastly green tinge. Most people think chlorine is the culprit, but it's more likely copper that causes the color change. Oxidized metals in the water bind to the protein in the hair shaft and deposit their color. The metal that produces the green tint is copper, which is most commonly found in algicides, which many people use in their swimming pools. If your child's hair turns green, you can get the color out by using a clarifying shampoo (see page 54). The best thing to do is prevent the copper from binding to the hair by sealing the hair cuticle with a conditioner before swimming, or (even better) wearing a rubber swim cap. Rinsing the hair immediately after leaving the pool will help, too.

## Static Cling

Hair tends to get charged up, especially during the winter when the air is dry and your child is pulling hats and earmuffs on to stay warm. If her hair becomes flyaway—or sticks to her head in a clump from static cling—simply reach for a fabric softener sheet (the kind you use in the clothes dryer) and rub it lightly over her head. Or rub in a dime-sized amount of a light styling cream to calm things down. If hair is curly or wavy, mist with water and scrunch.

## Hat Hair

Kids need hats to keep warm in cold winter months—or for playing sports in the summer—but they can make hair look flat or oddly indented once they're removed. To give hair a boost, either gently use your fingertips to fluff hair at the roots, or flip the hair upside down and brush it to add volume back in.

## Split Ends

When hair is damaged and dry from going too long between trims or overuse of heated styling aids, the ends literally split in two, giving hair a fuzzy look. Conditioners will smooth things out temporarily (kind of like gluing the hair back together), but they won't repair the damage. The best thing you can do is go for a trim to remove those splits before they spread higher up the strand. As a rule, trim hair every four to six weeks to keep it healthy.

## Dull Hair

Your child's once-glossy hair has lost its sheen . . . and you're not sure how or why. The culprit is likely a buildup of products that are now coating the hair shaft, making it look dull and dingy. A clarifying shampoo (see page 54) will help remove the buildup. Once the shine returns, use the shampoo once a week to keep hair glistening.

## Lice

It's the four-letter word that parents dread most: Lice is probably the biggest hair crisis you will confront when it comes to your kids. Just the thought of it makes most parents cringe—and start scratching. Head lice are common and affect up to 12 million kids each year in all socioeconomic groups. Most schools do lice checks, and unfortunately, it's common to get a call saying, "Your kid has lice." Don't panic. Your child is probably already upset about having bugs in her hair. Also, the diagnosis may not be correct. Sometimes children have dandruff that resembles nits (lice eggs), or dead or empty nits that are not in their normal position against the scalp. If you think your child has lice but you don't actually *see* any live lice, see your pediatrician to confirm the diagnosis.

### The Facts of Lice
#### How do they get it?
Kids between the ages of five and twelve get lice because of the way they play. Sharing hats, helmets, and clothing are all easy ways to spread these crawly creatures. Contrary to popular belief, lice do not jump or fly. Lice crawl and are usually transmitted by direct head-to-head contact with any infested people or their belongings. Lice are highly contagious and can spread quickly from person to person, especially in group settings (such as schools, childcare centers, slumber parties, locker rooms, and camps).

Head lice have nothing to do with lack of cleanliness; your child isn't dirty if she gets lice. In fact, lice prefer clean, healthy heads! They can live on a head for about thirty days, and in the environment (on pillows or clothes) for up to forty-eight hours.

### Can I do anything to prevent it?

The best way to prevent lice is to educate your child about how not to get them. Don't freak her out, just inform her. Teach her never to share hats, scarves, hair accessories, brushes, or combs—not even if she's playing dress-up with friends. It's a good idea to also occasionally clean things your child's head frequently touches, such as pillows, sleeping bags, car seats, and headphones.

Beyond that, tea tree oil is touted as a great treatment for preventing head lice. Use an all-natural, tea tree oil–based shampoo and conditioner every other day. As an alternative, add tea tree oil to your usual shampoo and wash hair with it every other day, or mix tea tree oil with water in a spray bottle and mist your child's hair before she heads out for the day. Also consider lightly spraying pillowcases, hoods, or hats as a preventive measure.

### How do I know if she has it?

The main symptom of head lice infestation is itching, particularly around the ears, back of neck, and crown. This comes from the bites of the lice, and if your child scratches too much, these bites can become infected. If that's the case, they may appear red or crusty, and may even cause swollen lymph glands in your child's neck (which may require antibiotics). But sometimes your child won't be itchy; it depends on how sensitive her skin is to the lice. It can sometimes take weeks for kids with lice to start scratching. Even if she doesn't have symptoms, it's a good idea to check your child's hair regularly (at least once a week)—especially because these pests are very hard to spot. If there is an outbreak in her class or school, be especially diligent.

Lice are the size of a sesame seed and are light brown in color. Nits are tiny (the size of a grain of sugar, smaller than a pinhead), white-to-light-gray eggs that attach to one side of the hair shaft and do not come off easily—the key difference between nits and dandruff or dried hair product.

Follow these steps for a thorough check; a magnifying glass and bright light may help you see nits better, but lice will run from the light (and can hinder your search).

- Part hair in a straight line down the back of the head to view the most scalp area.

- Look for live lice and also their eggs, or nits. Nits are a teardrop shape and have a pearly shine and always lie on only one side of the hair shaft.

- Repeat part behind ears vertically as well as horizontally, checking in sections.

- If you think you see a nit, run your finger over it. A nit will feel hard like a shell and will not move. It feels tightly glued onto the hair shaft.

If you find something suspicious, and you're not 100 percent sure it's lice or nits, take your child to the pediatrician.

## Treating Lice

The most effective treatment is the old-fashioned method of combing hair with a special lice comb and conditioner, and painstakingly removing nits/lice manually. It's also the least harmful method. There are places that specialize in this kind of removal; they can be pricey but they are the best way to get rid of lice.

FDA-approved treatments include both over-the-counter and prescription drugs in the form of shampoos, creams, and lotions (such as Rid or Nix), but many of these products are not for use on children under the age of two, so read the label carefully before using any on your child. Recently, the FDA approved a new prescription medication for the treatment of head lice. Ulesfia Lotion (benzyl alcohol 5 percent) is approved for use on children six months of age and older.

If your child is very young, or you're worried about chemical treatments, there are other natural and alternative approaches to ridding hair of lice—like smothering lice with olive oil, mayonnaise, Vaseline, or conditioner. Before you try them, talk to your pediatrician to determine what will work best for you and your child. Also note that these treatments may be very difficult to wash out of the hair.

Occasionally, you may come across lice that are stubborn and don't respond to treatment. There are salon and at-home services that can help you de-louse, and also medications for resistant lice (such as Ovide, Lindane, Bactrim, Ivermectim, or Elimite).

Again, your family doctor is your best advisor. And once the lice themselves are killed, you will also have to patiently and diligently remove nits with a lice comb, an extremely fine-tooth comb often made of metal. The purpose of the extra-fine teeth is to remove the nits or lice.

Remember that lice treatment isn't just about clean hair. You'll need to disinfest all your child's combs and brushes by soaking them in hot water (at least 130°F) for 5 to 10 minutes. Machine wash and dry clothing, bed linens, stuffed animals, and other items using hot water (130°F) and a high-heat drying cycle. Clothing and items that are not washable can be dry-cleaned or sealed in a plastic bag and stored for two weeks. Vacuum the floor and furniture, particularly where your child was sitting, playing, or lying in the past 48 hours. Head lice survive less than two days if they fall off the scalp. Finally, don't forget to check everyone in your family, even a week after your child has finished treatment, to make sure everyone is clear.

## Dear Cozy,

*My daughter came home from sleepaway camp with lice—does this mean that we need to treat her two siblings and my husband and me as well?*

*Just because your daughter has lice, it doesn't mean the whole family will have it—especially if you treat it quickly and efficiently. Only those with a proven infestation should be treated, although everyone should be checked daily to weekly.*

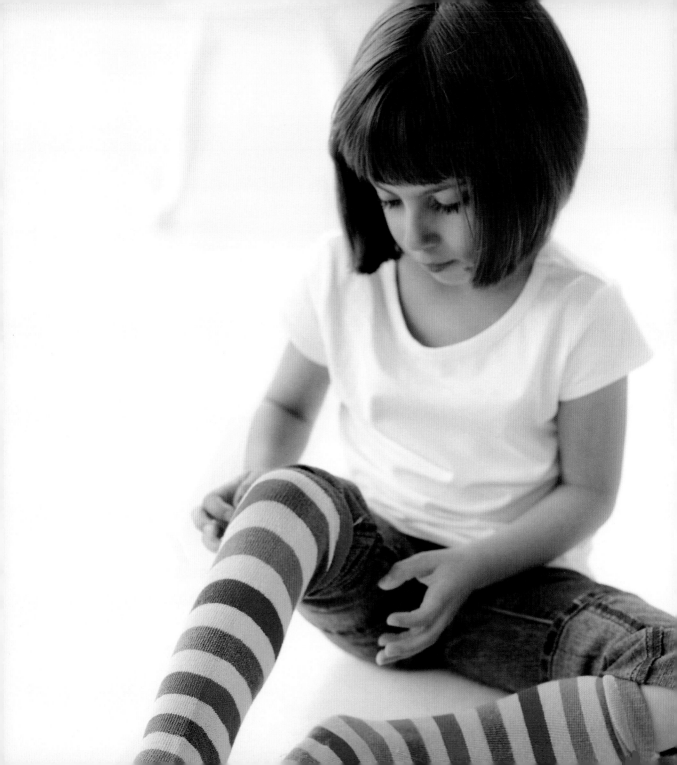

# CHAPTER 7

# Cool
# Cuts

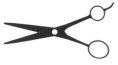

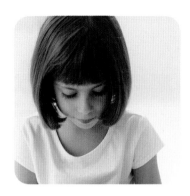

***It takes some*** time—and talking—to get to the point where you're truly comfortable putting your hair in someone else's hands. The same goes for your child; she's also probably worried about what her hair will look like when the stylist is done. Will her hair come out right? Will it be too short? There are several things you can do to ensure both of you get exactly what you want.

Before you decide on a hairdo, do your homework. Check out parenting or teen magazines and tear out lots of pictures of kids' styles you and your child like, to show to your stylist (you can even bring this book with you as a reference). A picture tells a thousand words. Use one whole look or the bangs from one, the length from another, and the sides from yet another picture. Ask the stylist's opinion whether these cuts will add up to a feasible look. Don't forget to let your child have some input. She'll feel more at ease and part of the process if she can explain what hairstyles she likes or doesn't like.

Be realistic about the style you are choosing. Are you choosing a straight hairstyle for your wavy-haired daughter? The stylist may be good . . . but she's not a miracle worker! If you don't find a photo of exactly what you want, make a list of what you are looking for. Is it versatility? A look that's neat and tidy and easy to care for? Or something a little more grown-up for your child's first day at a new school? Write down adjectives to describe your ideal look: cute, simple, soft, sweet, etc.

When you get to the salon, be extremely specific! The words *trim* or *cut* mean different things to different people. Rather than say "trim my daughter's hair," show the length of hair you'd like to cut off or the desired length of the final haircut with your fingers (see "What's an inch?" below) when hair is dry. Be sure to discuss your routine with the stylist so he/she understands your needs. Are you willing to spend twenty minutes blow-drying your child's hair, or do you just want to brush and go in the morning? Also let the stylist know of any challenges regarding your child's hair. This may influence the cut he/she gives, and may also help the stylist give you advice. Before the cut begins, ask the stylist to paraphrase back to you what he/she heard and make sure you're both on the same page.

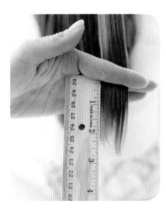

## What's an inch?

When you're telling your stylist how much to snip, show length with your fingers, rather than saying a number on a ruler.

## Shape Smarts

Here's a little secret that all hairstylists know: The shape of your face—not your hair texture—is the best guide for what cut will be the most flattering. If you're not sure of the shape of your child's face (sometimes it's tough to tell), clip or tie back her hair and have her look in a mirror while you trace the shape of her hairline and jaw with a lip or eye pencil. (You can let her draw in the smiley face when you're done!) Keep in mind that a child's face shape changes as she matures.

*Oval* The length of the face is equal to one and a half times the width.
**Best cuts:** This is a versatile face shape; almost any cut will look great.
**Worst cuts:** Heavy bangs or shaggy styles that hang in the face, obscuring its shape.

**Round** The face is as wide as it is long; your child may have apple cheeks or a rounded chin.
**Best cuts:** Full styles that have height at the crown; cute flips, wispy bangs, fringy cuts that angle in toward the face.
**Worst cuts:** Chin-length hair that is rounded like the face (such as a bob); this will make the face appear wider.

*Heart-Shaped* Your child has wide cheekbones and/or forehead and a narrow jaw, tapering to a point at the chin.
**Best cuts:** A classic chin-length bob—especially a swingy one—looks great because it shows off those fabulous cheekbones. Side-parted styles and side-swept bangs also work well.
**Worst cuts:** Too-short styles, which will make the chin look pointy.

*Square* The forehead and jaw line widths are close to equal (with a broad, straight forehead and an angular jaw).
**Best cuts:** Any style that softens the angles of her face: soft waves, wispy layers, and bangs. Short to medium lengths look best.
**Worst cuts:** Too-straight styles or anything very sleek or severe.

## Bang Basics

Little girls like the look of bangs, but parents worry that hair will always be in their eyes. The trick is to keep them trimmed. Bangs can jazz up a basic style, because they give so much versatility. You can sweep them back or to the side; wear them straight or choppy, or even pull just a few playful fringes forward. Just keep in mind that, once you cut them, you're stuck with them for a while.

Bangs work for most hair types, even curly or wavy, but it's a good idea to avoid them if your child's hair or skin is oily; bangs can promote acne on the forehead.

*Blunt bangs* are worn just above the eyebrow and cut precisely straight across, from one side to the other.

*Side bangs* are long or short fringes that are angled to be swept off to the side of the face rather than covering the forehead.

*Feathered bangs* are lighter and more textured than other bangs; the stylist actually cuts into them at different angles, so they appear slightly jagged and thinner at the ends, like the edges of a feather. They can be worn across the forehead or swept to the side. Feathered bangs are good for all hair types. For thick hair, feathering the bangs will help bangs look less blunt. For finer hair, feathered bangs can help add a more textured look.

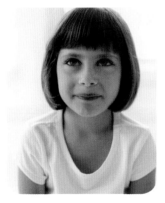
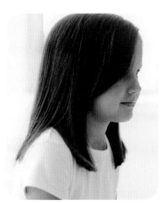
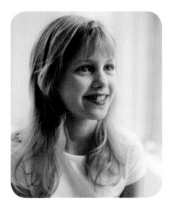

Blunt bangs      Side bangs      Feathered bangs

**Dear Cozy,**

*My daughter was dying for bangs . . . and now, a month later, she hates them. How do we grow them out?*

*I'm sorry to say there's no instant or easy way to erase her bangs. You both have to be patient; they're not permanent, and they will (I promise!) eventually grow out, although there may be a short time when the hair looks a little awkward. Pulling the hair back with cute, cool accessories will distract the eye from the bangs and help hide the problem. It will likely take six months to a year to completely grow them out, but your daughter—and you—may be surprised to find a style along the way that you actually like, like side bangs (see page 84). It's also a good idea to consult a professional stylist during the growing-out process to help blend the hair and make recommendations.*

## DIY Haircuts

Yes, you can cut your child's hair—and it can save you time and money. These basic trims—for bangs and common kid cuts—are easy enough to do at home. Straight hair is easier to cut than curly hair; very curly locks may require a pro to shape them properly. But if you're willing to give it a go, cover your child in a smock or make sure she's wearing an old T-shirt that can go straight into the wash. Many people choose to trim their child's hair in the bath because of the easy cleanup, but you have less control in a slippery tub. It's easier to have your child sit in a chair in front of a DVD or other distraction (a video game, book, or toy should do the trick).

While the hair is dry, decide on length. Don't rush—even if you're worried you're losing your audience. If you zip through this process, you're more likely to make mistakes (and there's no way to put hair back once you cut it off!). Plan to snip off a smaller amount than you think you want to trim. You can always go back later and cut more. When you're done, check your work carefully; comb the hair out to make sure the lines are even and snip away any stray strands. And always be mindful that your child may move suddenly—so be prepared: Watch where you hold your scissors and keep combs or blades safely away from eyes. If you're cutting close to the eyes (such as for bangs), give your child a little warning to stay superstill while you snip!

## Wet or Dry?

Haircutting can be done on either wet or dry hair—and most stylists have a personal preference. Some people like to do quick trims (such as bangs or wisps) dry because it allows them to see where the hair falls naturally (wetting hair weighs it down and makes it appear longer than it does when dry). On the other hand, wet hair tends to stick together, which makes it slightly more manageable when you need to do a precise cut (small pieces won't slip away from your blades). Most parents find it easier to cut hair wet for this reason. It need only be damp, not drenched.

## The Right Scissors

If you're going to be cutting hair at home, be sure to invest in a good pair of haircutting scissors or barber shears, available in beauty supply stores. Scissors with pointed blades that are 5½ to 6 inches in length are the best for trimming. Never use manicure scissors or the ones from your sewing kit! Haircutting scissors are beveled so they cut down and through the hair cleanly, while other scissors will push the hair forward into clumps (translation: you'll wind up with a crooked cut). Also, be sure to take proper care of your scissors: Wipe them down after use with a soft cloth and store them in a pouch or case so they don't get nicked or bent.

## What You'll Need

Cape or smock to put over your child

Newspapers, a garbage bag, or
  a disposable plastic tablecloth
  to spread under the chair where
  you're cutting, for easier cleanup

Wide-tooth comb

Spray bottle with water

Fine-tooth comb

Several large butterfly clips

Barber scissors

# Trimming Bangs

*These instructions are for blunt bangs. For other types of bangs, see the variations on page 83.*

**Step 1:** Using a wide-tooth comb, part the hair down the middle.

**Step 2:** Mist hair lightly with water and comb through to remove tangles.

**Step 3:** Measure along the part about an inch from the hairline, and use the fine-tooth comb to draw a line from that point to the edge of the hairline at the outer corner of one eyebrow, forming a triangle-shaped section of hair. Clip this section away from the rest, and repeat on the other side of the part (illus. 1). Clip the rest of the hair away from these two bang sections. If your child's hair is fine, you may want to start ½ inch from the hairline instead of a full inch.

**Step 4:** Comb the two bang sections of hair straight down in front of the face.

**Step 5:** With your fingers, separate the center inch of the bang and hold it down toward the nose between your pointer and middle fingers just below the eyebrows (illus. 2). Don't twist it; be sure to hold it loosely, not taut, or it will be too short after you cut it. Tell the child to close her eyes, so she doesn't get hair in them. With the other hand, hold the scissors straight and snip just below your fingers.

**Step 6:** Repeat this process with the section of bang on either side of the center one, using the length of the center section as your guide (illus. 3). Be sure to pull the hair straight down, not at an angle toward the center, or you'll end up with curved bangs (see page 83).

*Step 7:* Evaluate bangs after they dry and touch up if necessary.

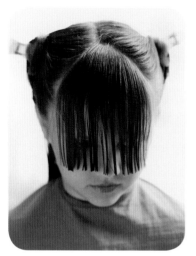

**1**

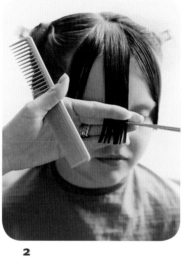

**2**

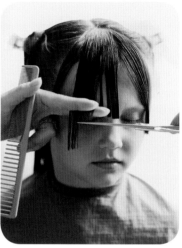

**3**

*If you want the bangs to be slightly layered and less chunky, trim as for blunt bangs, then comb the entire bang straight up vertically and trim it again, using the shortest hair length as your guide.*

*For wispy bangs, trim the bangs as described on pages 81 and 82, then hold the bangs about an inch from the ends between your pointer and middle fingers. With the other hand, hold the scissors perpendicular to the edge of the hair, and use just the tips to snip little V-shaped sections about ⅛ inch into the bangs. This will make them look jagged.*

*Curved bangs are shorter in the center and longer on the sides; they curve slightly around the face. Cut the center section first as for blunt bangs. Instead of pulling the side sections straight down, pull them at an angle toward the center section and cut straight across the angle to match the length of the center section. When you release the hair, the outer two sections will be slightly longer at the temples.*

# Basic Blunt Cut

*Use this for straight, wavy, or curly hair that's one length all around.*

**Step 1:** Mist hair and comb through to detangle. Section the hair as described on page 59. The two bottom sections will serve as your guide. Once you cut this hair to length, you will match all other section lengths to it.

**Step 2:** Be sure the child is looking down, with her eyes on her knees, chin slightly down. This is especially important for girls who have long hair. Doing this will ensure the best cutting angle and keep the bottom layer from being longer than the top layer. Keeping her head in one position throughout will also ensure an even cut. Comb out a small section of hair at the part (approximately an inch in width) and hold it between your pointer and middle finger right above the length you want to remove (illus. 1). Hold the scissors straight and the hair taut, then guide the blades of the scissors straight beneath your fingers as you snip.

**Step 3:** Using the length of this center section as a guide, work your way out on either side of it, separating and cutting small sections of hair in the same way so they all match the length of the first section (illus. 2).

**Step 4:** Once you're done cutting the two bottom sections, section out 1 inch of hair along the bottom of the sections still in the clips and continue cutting in the same way, 1-inch section by 1-inch section, until all hair is trimmed (illus. 3). For each new section, comb the hair, then cut it to match the length of the first section. Comb the side sections straight down toward the floor, not back behind the ears, and match the length of the back sections.

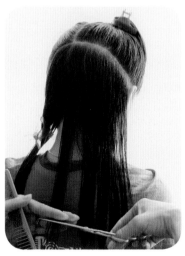
1

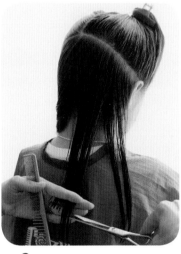
2

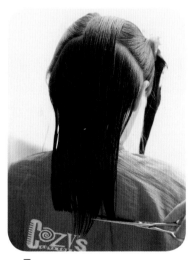
3

## VARIATION

*Cutting curly hair is a little more challenging. Beware of shrinkage! Curly hair will bounce up much shorter than you estimate—as much as 3 inches—when you trim it. And you're also pulling it straighter to cut it. For a rough guide of how much hair will shrink, measure hair when it's dry versus when it's wet. That way you know how much you really want to trim—it may be less than you think!*

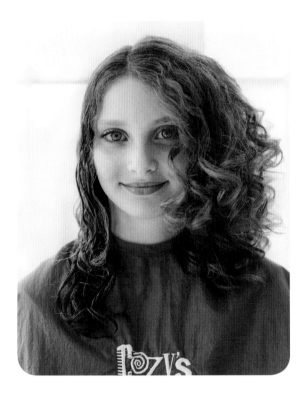

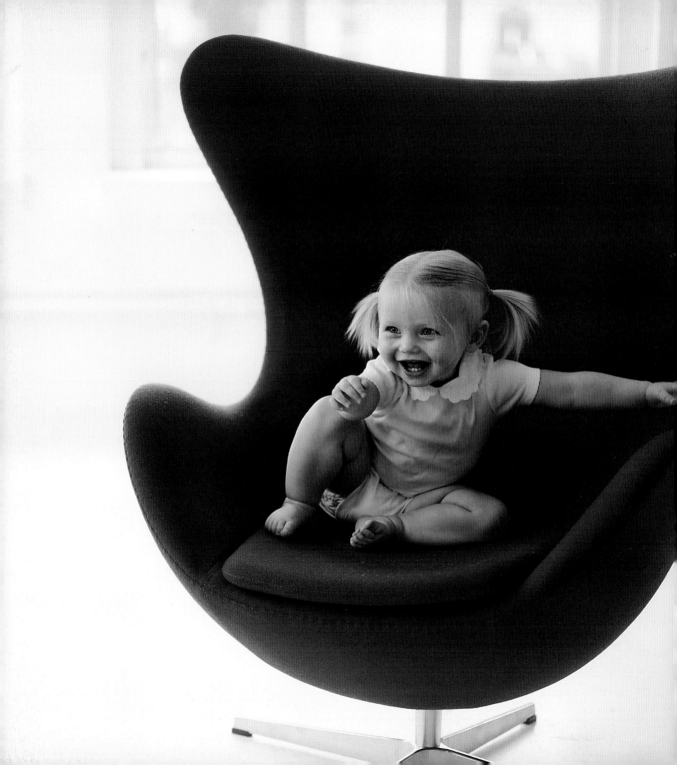

CHAPTER 8

# Baby Hair Care

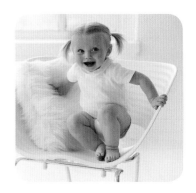

**Even if your** baby remains relatively bald during the first year of life (see page 93), it is still important to keep her scalp clean to encourage healthy hair growth.

You should care for baby's hair the same way you care for baby: gently and delicately, with lots of TLC. Avoid putting pressure on the soft spot on the top of the baby's head when you shampoo or brush. Most babies, and even kids up to the age of five, have a sensitive scalp. When washing the hair and the scalp of a baby or young child, be sure to go very slow and easy (don't scrub hard with your nails). And don't feel you need to wash her hair frequently; a baby's hair should be washed only when necessary (if it looks oily/dirty or has food in it).

Many pediatricians recommend the use of a baby shampoo (look for the words *baby shampoo* on the label) during the first years of an infant's life. Choose a baby shampoo that doesn't contain sulfates, the preservatives that are used in most adult hair care products, and they won't sting eyes. Additionally, baby shampoo contains milder cleansers than adult products and has a balanced pH, which is gentler on a baby's sensitive scalp.

After washing, gently towel-dry baby's hair and then (if it's long enough) brush it into place with a baby brush (these have softer bristles that won't scratch the scalp).

## The First Cut

A child's first haircut is a milestone; there's a reason baby books have a page dedicated to this event! It's time for the first haircut when the hair starts to get in your baby's eyes, is bothersome on the back of her neck, or when flyaways on the sides start to look like wings. Many people resist baby's first haircut because they want the hair to grow longer. The truth is, with a teeny cleanup around the ends, the hair will look much healthier, thicker, and neater.

However, as with any new experience, a first haircut can be very frightening for a young child (and traumatic for parents!). One two-year-old even asked her mom if hair bleeds when it gets cut . . . like her finger! There's a lot you can do to nip your child's fears about that first snip and make it fun.

Familiarity makes anything less scary. Bring your child with you when *you* go for your haircut. She'll be able to watch the process and it will be less intimidating once it's her turn. When the time comes, take her to the salon where she'll have her haircut prior to the day of the appointment. It's good to let kids see other kids having a haircut (and surviving!) so they know not to be scared. You can even play-act hair salon with dolls—let your child pretend to be the stylist and give dolly a new do!

Language can also help remove fear from the process. When talking to a child about a haircut, you might want to use another word such as *trim* or *style*. *Cut* can be a scary word because children always hear it in a negative context. Use nicknames for some of the equipment that can frighten children. For example, call the blow-dryer "the wind machine" or the scissors "snippies."

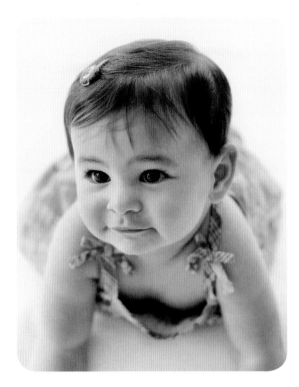

The first cut doesn't have to come with tears and tantrums! Distraction is the key. If your child is busy, she won't be crying or whimpering. Most kids' salons will have fun seats, toys, and DVDs to keep them mesmerized while the stylist quickly snips away. If you're not going to a kids' salon, bring your own bag of tricks—for example, a book, bubbles, a favorite toy, or a lollipop. Bringing a snack or treat or a bottle/sippy cup is also a good idea. And if your baby squirms in the chair, let her sit on your lap instead. Just cuddling Mommy or Daddy can keep her calm and content.

Finally, there are practical considerations. If you are not taking your child to a children's-only salon, make sure you request a stylist who has experience with and likes working with children. Make the appointment in advance so you know the receptionist is not just putting you in with whoever is free. Schedule the appointment for a time of day that is good for your child—not before naptime or at a time of day when she is tired or cranky. Also, bring a change of shirt in case your child doesn't want to wear the salon cape.

Remember to relax. If you are nervous, your child will sense it right away. Most important, try to enjoy it. Don't forget your camera! Don't forget to save the first lock of hair! You may want to bring a small plastic bag to put it in.

## Does Baby's Hair Cause Mom Heartburn?

**Researchers at Johns Hopkins think this old wives' tale is true: They surveyed a group of mothers and found that 82 percent of those who had moderate or severe heartburn during pregnancy gave birth to a baby with an average or above-average amount of hair. Most of the women who didn't have heartburn gave birth to a baby with little or no hair.**

## Baby's Bad Hair Days

*Untamable Tresses* Your baby has crazy curls or a stubborn cowlick that simply won't obey, no matter how you attempt to brush, smooth, or calm them. This is probably because the chemical bonds that give hair its texture are still developing in a child's first year. Don't stress; hair usually settles down by age one.

*Cradle Cap* If your baby's scalp has a thick yellow or brown scaling or crusting, it's most likely cradle cap. The cause of cradle cap is not known, but it is not caused by an infection, an allergy, or poor hygiene. Experts believe it is the normal buildup of sticky skin oils and sloughed skin cells. This is very common, especially in newborns, and usually clears up on its own in six to twelve months. Baby is probably not even bothered by it, but if it bothers you, shampoo more frequently and gently brush your baby's scalp with a soft brush or a washcloth. Some parents rub a dot of natural oil, such as almond or olive oil, into the baby's scalp and leave it on for about 10 minutes, then gently comb the scaly flakes from the scalp with a fine comb. Follow with a gentle baby shampoo and rinse well.

**Baldness** About a third of babies are born with no hair at all. Though it seems like a long time to wait—especially when you have a girl—most babies grow plenty of hair by their first birthday. Until then, there is nothing you can do to speed hair growth along. There is a common misconception that shaving a baby's head will make hair grow in faster and thicker, but hair is dead keratin pushed out by hair follicles under the skin (see page 4) and cutting or shaving hair on the surface cannot affect cell growth beneath the skin.

## Dear Cozy

*My baby was born with a gorgeous head of thick hair . . . and she now has several bald patches! Is this normal?*

*Baldness is a very common problem for babies. Experts suspect that a newborn's hormone levels drop right after birth, which can cause her to lose much of the hair she was born with. Many babies today develop balding on the back of their heads from being continually placed on their backs to sleep (to decrease the risk of SIDS). If this is the case for your baby, simply give her more "tummy time" when she's awake. There are other conditions that cause hair loss—including medical ones like thyroid conditions or fungal infections—but they're very uncommon in children under twelve months old. If you're still concerned, ask your pediatrician.*

## Cute Styles for Small Fries

If you have a girl, it can be hard to resist cute hair accessories. But keep in mind a few safety guidelines. Tiny clips are a choking hazard for children under the age of three, and since baby hair is fine, a clip can easily fall out and wind up in your baby's mouth or poke her in the eye. Make sure the hair accessories you choose stay firmly in place (see if you can tug them out easily). If not, save them only for photo ops when you're keeping a watchful eye.

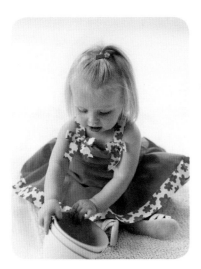

**Cutie-Pie Clip** Even if your baby daughter doesn't have a lot of hair, you can still give her some style. Avoid the comb-over look by allowing baby bangs to fall gently over the forehead. Most babies will pull out whatever you place in the hair (although some are certainly born fashionistas and don't seem to mind). It's harder for them to remove a small elastic, and you can always put a cute clip over it. Also, the faster you are able to put baby's hair in a clip or an elastic, the less likely she is to notice and/or pull it out.

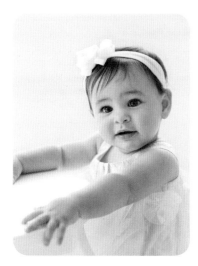

**Baby Band** A stretchy headband is an easy option, especially if your child doesn't have lots of locks yet—or has none at all! A headband is pretty and feminine, plus it's soft and comfy. If baby protests as you put it on, make a game of it. And again, be sure not to leave baby wearing it unattended, such as during naps; a stretchy band can also be a strangulation hazard.

## Dear Cozy,

*Can I use my adult shampoo and conditioner on my child?*

*I highly recommend that children use hair products that are specifically formulated for the different needs of children's hair. A respectable children's formulation will have vitamins and minerals that will be absorbed into the hair and are great for growing children. Also, these products tend to be a little lighter (won't weigh down hair) and gentler (tear-free) for children. Lastly, I recommend looking for products that are paraben-free (see page 57), since the jury is still out on the safety of parabens in beauty products.*

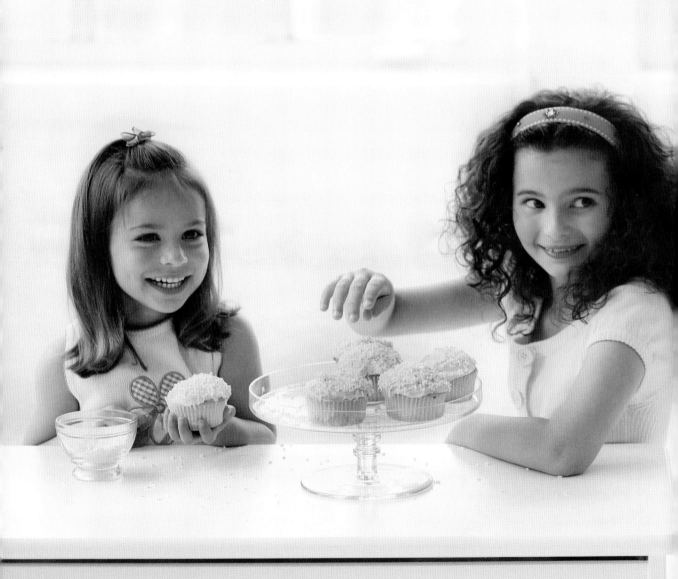

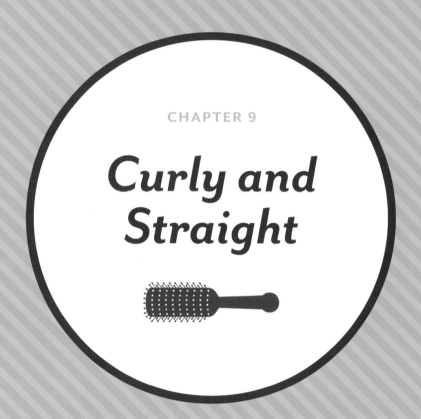

CHAPTER 9

# *Curly and Straight*

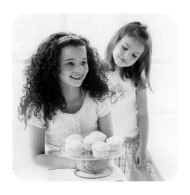

***Superstraight and supercurly*** hair are both uniquely wonderful and uniquely challenging! Your child may not love what she was born with and may beg you to help her change it: We all get envious from time to time of what we don't have. There's certainly nothing wrong with occasionally granting your girl's hair fantasy (that's what styling tools were made for—see chapter 3 for the best tools to use). But you should encourage your child to love doing what comes naturally with her straight or curly hair rather than trying to coax it into submission. It will work wonders for her self-esteem—and make both of your lives a whole lot easier. The styles in this chapter are especially for straight and curly hair types, although all will work fine with wavy hair, too.

## Curly Girl

**The good news:** Her hair has natural volume and texture: instant glam. Curls can range from tight ringlets to zigzag waves.

**The bad news:** The biggest problem is that it gets knotted, matted, and frizzy and can be torture to brush. It can look wild and crazy if not cared for correctly.

Caring for curly hair is more of a challenge than caring for straight. For starters, NEVER brush curly hair! Brushing the hair will make it look fuzzy. Comb curly hair with a wide-tooth comb when it is wet, to detangle it. Try doing this when your child is in the tub with conditioner in her hair. Wring the excess water out of her hair with your hands, then use a towel to gently blot out extra moisture. Part the damp hair and, using a nickel-sized amount of a styling product (such as an alcohol-free gel), scrunch the hair from tips to roots.

You also want to let curly hair air-dry. Don't blow-dry it unless you use a diffuser (see page 28), but keep in mind that most kids won't hold still that long; it takes much longer than a regular blow-dry. Using a blow-dryer without the diffuser will frizz, knot, and dry out curls, turning them into what one mom refers to as a "bird's nest."

A great haircut will help to enhance the curls. Layers are usually recommended. Products created specifically for curly hair truly do work to enhance the natural curl as well as keep hair from frizzing. The trick is to find the product that works best for your child's hair. There are many different types of products on the market (gels, waxes, serum, styling cream) and different people have different preferences as to what works best. For kids, try a basic alcohol-free gel, which holds the shape of the curl well and prevents frizz.

> ### Dear Cozy,
>
> *My daughter's curly hair always looks so dried out. What can I do?*
>
> *Keeping hair hydrated is critical to healthy curls. Here's a secret weapon: Do not rinse out all the conditioner. Leave in a little to add some extra moisture by doing a quick rather than thorough rinse. During the week, use a spray leave-in conditioner on the days in between shampooing.*

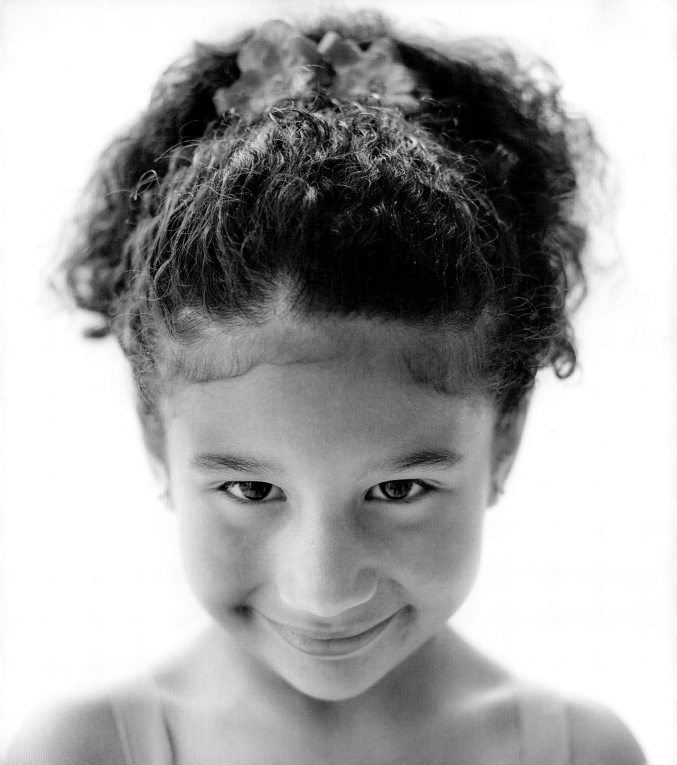

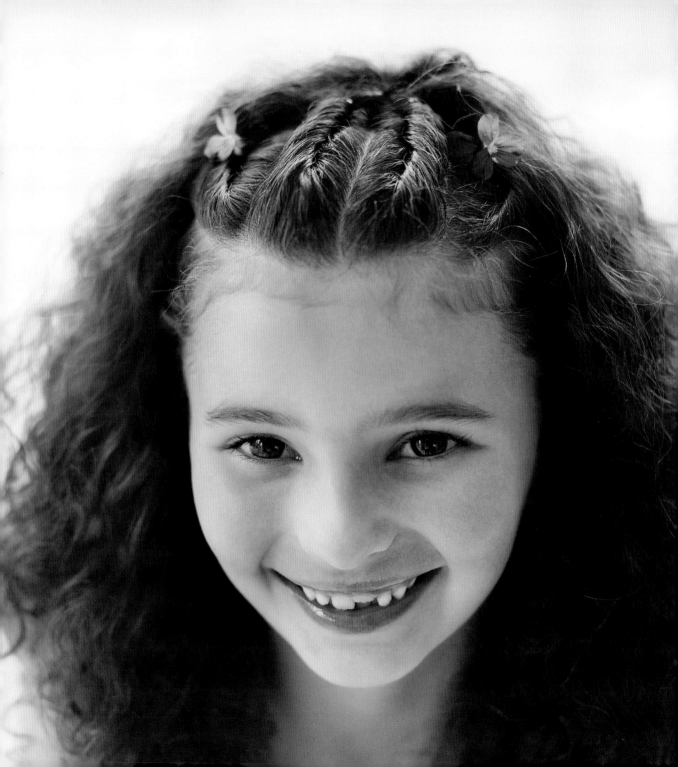

# The Quadruple Twist

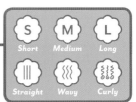

S — Short
M — Medium
L — Long

||| Straight
))) Wavy
$$$ Curly

*A quick flick of the wrist creates this cute coif that only looks complicated. You can fancy it up with pretty beads or barrettes.*

## What You'll Need

Spray bottle of water
Fine-tooth comb
Hair clip to section hair
Small ponytail holders
Mini–butterfly clips

Hair gel or light styling cream

**Time:**
10 minutes

**Step 1:** Mist the hair with the spray bottle to make it damp but not wet. Part it in the middle with a fine-tooth comb, and gather a section of hair on one side of the part, from the part to the outer eyebrow.

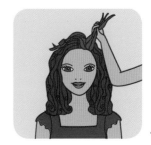

1

**Step 2:** Divide this section in half, with one half near the part and one half away from it (illus. 1). Clip the half closest to the part out of the way.

**Step 3:** Hold the remaining half and begin twisting it on a diagonal path toward the part. Twist firmly, gathering additional hair as you twist, but not so tightly that it hurts. Twist till you reach the part, then secure the end with a ponytail holder, letting the excess hair hang down (illus. 2).

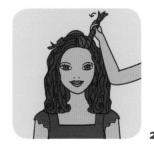

2

**Step 4:** Unclip the half-section closest to the part and mist again. Using the same method, twist this section firmly in the direction of the part. Secure with a ponytail holder.

**Step 5:** Repeat the process on the other side of the part to create two more twists, for a total of four (illus. 3).

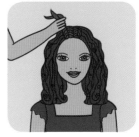

3

**Step 6:** Attach pretty mini–butterfly clips to the ponytail holder on each twist. Rub a pea-sized amount of gel or light styling cream between your palms and scrunch the curls to finish.

# Quarter Up

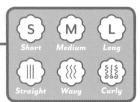

*This miniponytail style is great for a younger child; it keeps hair out of the eyes and looks sweet and playful.*

### What You'll Need
Brush

Ponytail holder, bow, clip,
  or scrunchie

**Time:**
10–20 minutes

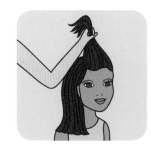

**Step 1:** Starting with dry hair, brush or comb it smooth and detangle it. Then brush or comb the hair straight back and lift a section off the crown, approximately eyebrow to eyebrow in width (see illus.). Pull the hair back no farther than 1.5 inches and to the side. Choosing how far back and how far off to the side will depend on the hair. For girls with shorter bangs, you may need to keep the hair closer to the hairline.

**Step 2:** Gather sectioned hair into a ponytail holder, bow, or scrunchie to create a miniponytail at the top of the head. For more volume, gather the ponytail more loosely to give the front of the hair a little height. Adorn with a fun ponytail holder or cute clip.

## Perfect Curls!

Every curly girl wants springy spirals—and you can grant that wish. This technique, however, will take a lot of work, so save it for special occasions. Start by shampooing and conditioning as usual. Blot hair with a towel and detangle with a wide-tooth comb. Apply a curl-enhancing spray or gel to damp hair and blow-dry with a diffuser to lift and separate curls. Once hair is completely dry, define curls using a curling iron. You'll be working in small sections (about 1 inch to 2 inches at a time). Wind the strand around the barrel of the iron, holding it there for only a few seconds. A larger barrel (1½ inches) will create longer, looser curls while a smaller barrel (¾ to 1 inch) will create tighter ringlets. When you've curled the entire head, allow the curls to cool, then finger-fluff (never brush!) to loosen them and make them more natural.

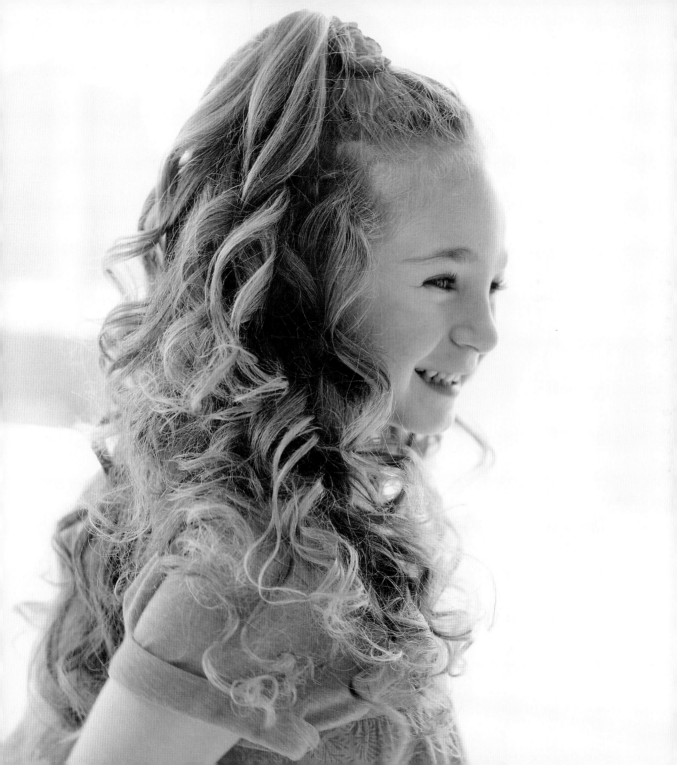

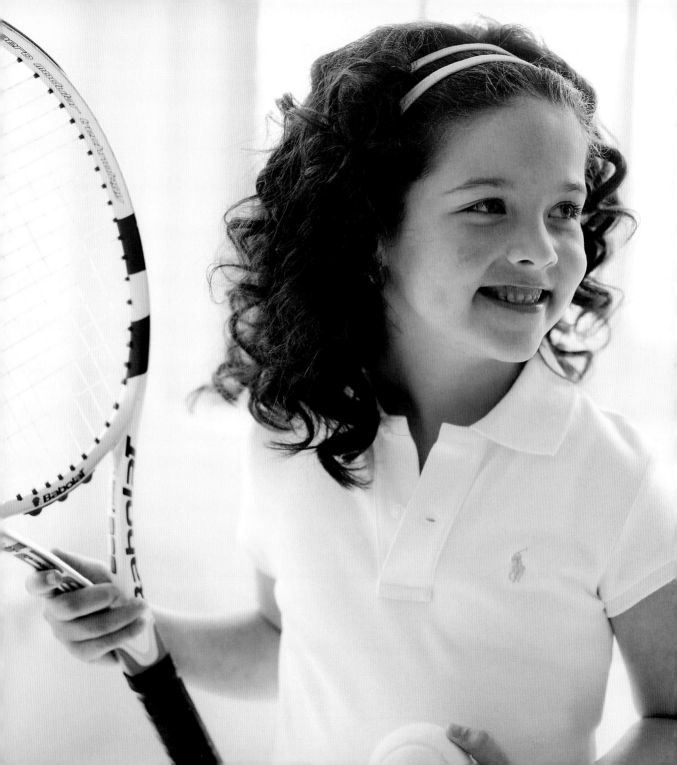

# Sporty Girl

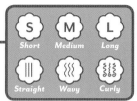

At home on the tennis courts or on the baseball field, this natural athlete needs a look that won't slow her down. This is a practical style for anytime you need to keep her hair out of her eyes.

## What You'll Need
Wide-tooth comb
Headband or terry sports band
Hair gel or light styling cream

**Time:**
Less than 5 minutes

**Step 1:** Starting with dry or damp hair, comb it smooth and detangle it. Now push a headband firmly back in the direction of the hair to keep it out of the eyes.

**Step 2:** Leave the rest of the hair natural. If hair is extra curly or wavy, rub a pea-sized amount of gel or light styling cream between your palms and scrunch the hair to finish.

### VARIATION
You could also make a ponytail or pigtails to get the hair off the neck, especially for outdoor play.

## *Straight Girl*

**The good news:** Her hair is naturally sleek and shiny; the layers of the cuticle lie flat and reflect light, making the hair glisten.

**The bad news:** Without special treatment, hair can look oily, dirty, or limp.

When washing your child's straight hair, use warm—not hot—water. The last rinse should be cooler, as cold water "seals" the hair by causing the cuticle to lie flat, making the hair look even shinier. Gently shampoo with a product formulated for your child's hair type. How often you shampoo depends on how oily the hair is (see page 21). Very oily hair should be washed every other day; normal to dry hair should be washed two to three times a week. Never use a brush (only a wide-tooth comb) on wet strands. Squeeze hair gently with a towel to get out the water; don't rub it. Straight hair is most fragile when it's wet.

Let hair air-dry as often as possible. Blow-dryers and styling tools can cause breakage. Avoid heavy hair products such as gels and waxes. These will weigh down straight hair, making it look limp—or worse, dirty. Mousse and light styling cream are better options. If hair needs a bit more volume, apply a dollop of mousse, and work it through the hair gently and evenly. Finally, trim the ends every four to six weeks to keep the hair neat-looking.

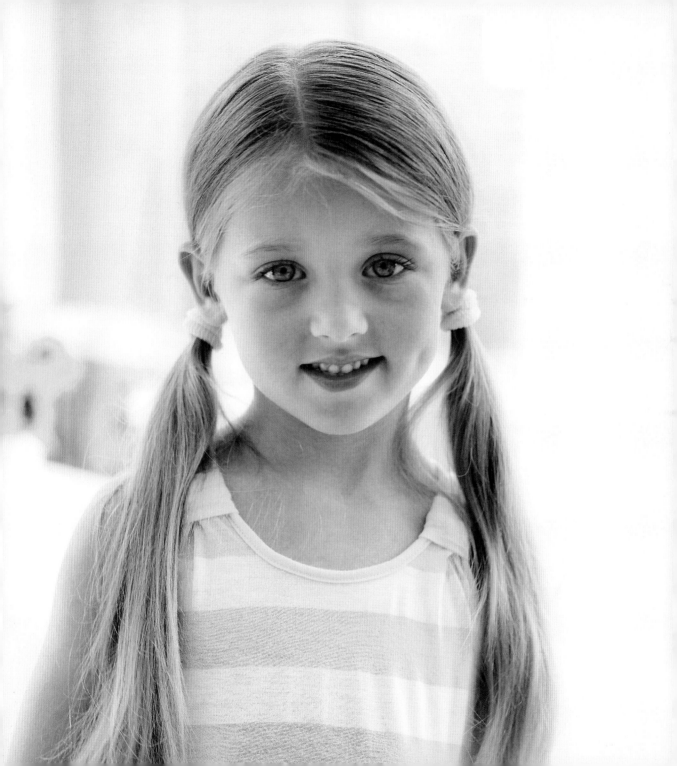

# Side Sweep

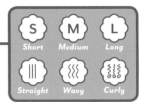

An easy style for straight hair—simply fasten with a fresh flower or a dazzling hair clip.

## What You'll Need

Paddle or round brush

Bobby pin or decorative barrette/
  mini–butterfly clip

Fresh flower (optional)

**Time:**

5 minutes

**Step 1:** Starting with dry hair, brush it smooth and detangle it. For more volume, you can wash or mist the hair and blow-dry using a round brush (for instructions, see page 116).

**Step 2:** Part the hair down the middle, or if you prefer, to one side. Using the brush and starting above the ear, sweep back a section of hair on one side and pin it up and back, anywhere above the ear that looks good.

**Step 3:** Tuck in a pretty bloom to cover the bobby pin—or use a decorative barrette or a mini–butterfly clip instead.

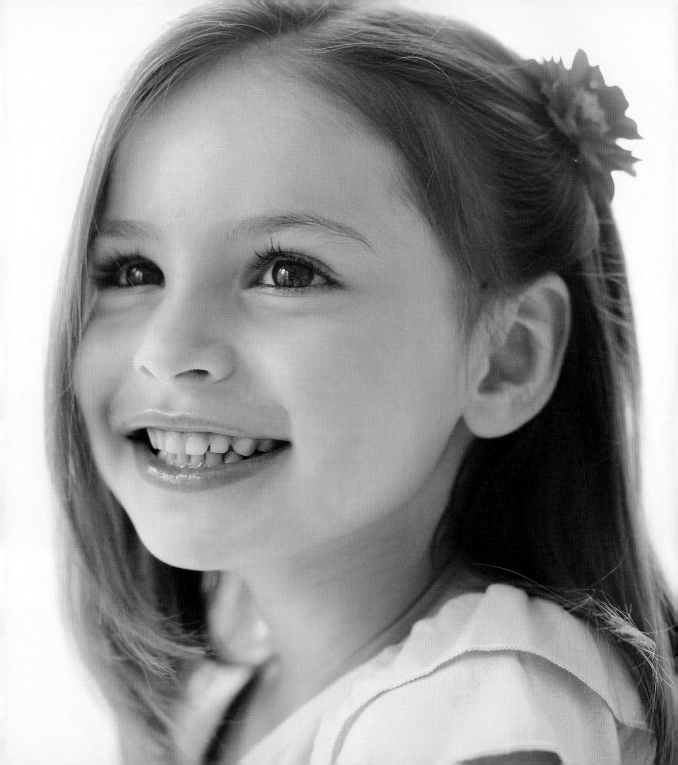

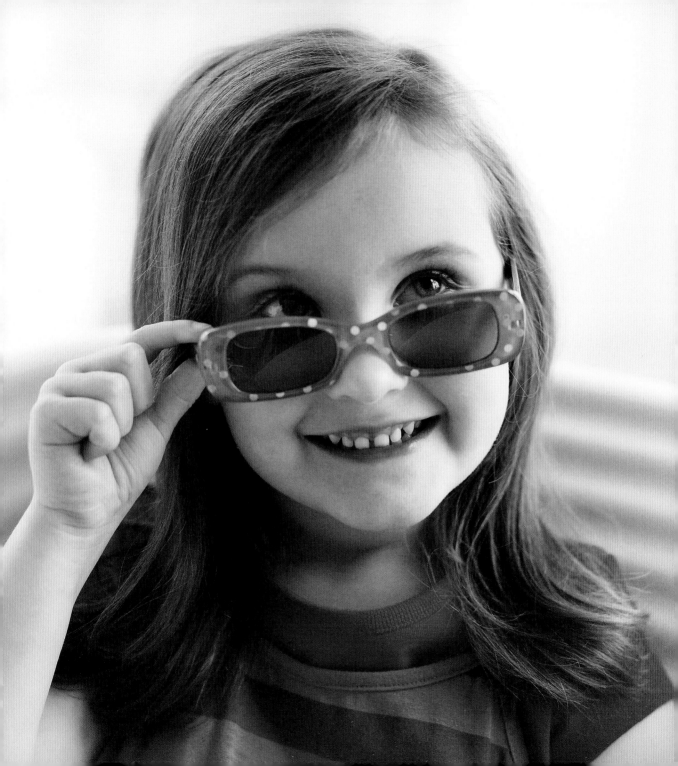

# Flipped Out!

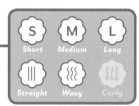

*So very retro, this style is a cute way to give a little sass to stick-straight strands. While you can try this look on any length hair, it works best on chin-length for a sharp, structured curve on the ends.*

### What You'll Need

Wide-tooth comb

Mousse or gel

Blow-dryer

Round brush

Curling iron

Hair spray

Cute clips (optional)

**Time:**

15 minutes

**Step 1:** Wash and condition hair as usual. Detangle with a wide-tooth comb and part to one side (or in the middle, if you prefer).

**Step 2:** Rub a quarter-sized amount of mousse or gel into the hair, distributing it evenly.

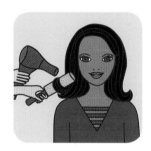

**Step 3:** Blow-dry hair, section by section, using a round brush (illus.) to give hair volume (for instructions, see page 116).

**Step 4:** When the hair is completely dry, use a curling iron just on the ends to flip them out and away from the face. If you wrap too much hair on the iron, you'll get a curl rather than that cool, curved edge. If hair is particularly stubborn and won't stay flipped out, try hot rollers on the ends (wrap hair just once and pin; see page 33) for a few minutes.

**Step 5:** Finish with a light mist of hair spray, and if you like, add some cute clips to accessorize.

# Glam Girl

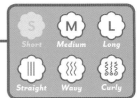

Hollywood, here she comes! This fantasy style will put stars in her eyes.

## What You'll Need

Paddle brush
Fine-tooth comb
Ponytail holder
Hair spray
Hairpins or hair clip

Thick headband, preferably glittery
  or sequined

**Time:**
10–15 minutes

**Step 1:** Starting with dry hair, brush it smooth and detangle it. Use the fine-tooth comb to section the hair from the top of one ear to the top of the other, creating a front section that will be teased. Use a ponytail holder to loosely pull back all the hair except this front section.

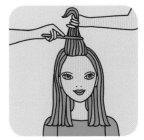

**1**

**Step 2:** Using a fine-tooth comb, back-comb the front section, from the ends toward the roots, teasing it to create volume (illus. 1). It will be easier if you work in small sections, 2 inches at a time.

**Step 3:** Once hair is teased, lightly brush it back and mist with hair spray. Secure it with pins or a clip at the back of the head (illus. 2).

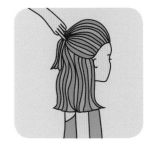

**2**

**Step 4:** Remove the ponytail holder from the rest of the hair, and slide on a sparkly headband, positioning it near the hairline to avoid flattening the teased section.

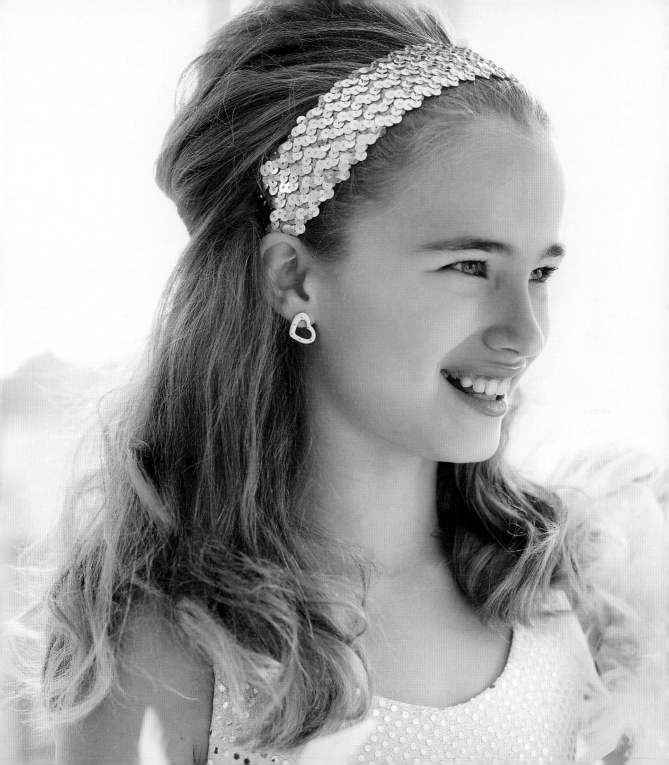

# Ready, Set, Blow!

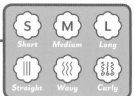

*A salon-quality blowout at home? It's absolutely possible. Just take your time, and remember that practice makes perfect. This technique can be used throughout the book where blow-drying is called for, and works best on medium to long hair.*

### What You'll Need

Wide-tooth comb
Leave-in conditioner
Mousse or light styling cream
  (optional)
Blow-dryer
Diffuser (optional)
Fine-tooth comb
Large butterfly clip

Brush: round to create volume, or a
  paddle brush for straightening and
  smoothing
Hair spray or shine spray

### Time:

15–30 minutes, depending on hair
  length

**Step 1:** Wash and condition hair as usual. Towel-dry; hair should be damp, not wet.

**Step 2:** Using a wide-tooth comb, detangle hair; apply leave-in conditioner (to protect hair from the heat of the dryer) and any other styling products desired, such as mousse or styling cream.

**Step 3:** For kids, it's best to use the coolest/lowest setting on your blow-dryer. If hair is still very wet, use the blow-dryer and your fingers to remove excess moisture before you start the blowout.

**Step 4:** Using a fine-tooth comb, section the hair following the directions on page 59. Clip the sides up and out of the way. Now select a section of hair at the back, 2–3 inches in width. Hold the dryer in one hand, the brush in the other.

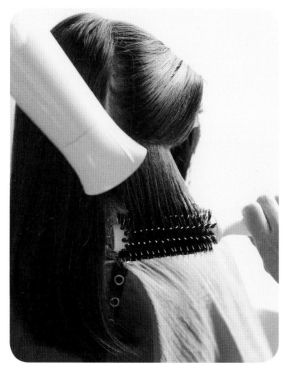

**Step 5:** Beginning at the roots (to avoid frizzing), use the brush to pull the section of hair taut. Start by drying the underside of the section, gently pulling the brush through to the ends, and lifting the hair out and away from the head.

**Step 6:** Once the underside is dry, point the nozzle of the dryer down onto the top side of the hair, at approximately a 45-degree angle toward you. This will smooth the cuticle and create shine. Again, use the brush to pull the section away from the head, stretching and straightening as you work from roots to ends.

**Step 7:** Continue slowly around the head, making sure each section is dry and straight before moving on to the next. Once you have finished the bottom, unclip the sides and work on them one at a time, starting at the ears and working toward the part.

**Step 8:** Finish with a light misting of hair spray or shine spray.

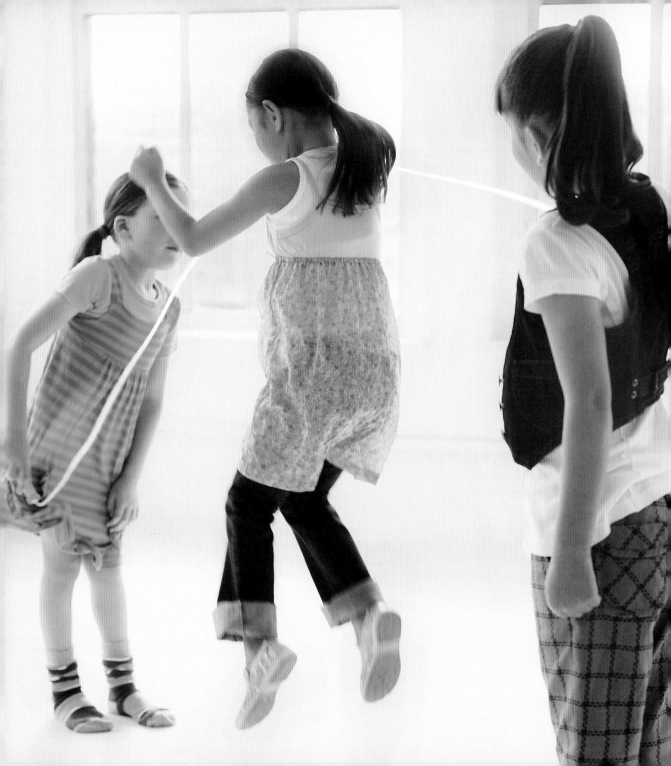

# CHAPTER 10

# Trendy Tails

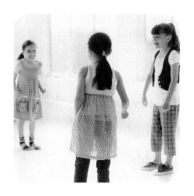

**Ponytails and pigtails** (a ponytail on each side of the head) are not just a popular style for girls, they're also mom-tested and -approved. They're a great way to keep hair neat, tidy, tangle-free, and out of the eyes during school and sports, and they work for absolutely every hair type. Anyone can execute the basics, but these styles have a bit more going for them. For a smoother look, spray hair with a light hair spray and gently comb in any flyaways with a fine-tooth comb after hair is in a ponytail.

Positioning the ponytail: High, low, in between, or on the sides? It's all up to you and your child—as well as the length of her hair.

- A low ponytail is great for shorter hair (so stray strands won't slip out). For low pigtails, part down the middle and gather the hair on each side behind the ear. Secure with a ponytail holder.

- High ponytails sit high on the head, or if you're doing high pigtails, above the ears. This is a great way to get superlong hair off your child's neck in the summer.

- A side ponytail can look a little softer, especially if hair is long enough to delicately drape over the shoulder. Gather all the hair loosely on one side, either below the ear or above it, and secure the ponytail with a pretty ponytail holder or scrunchie.

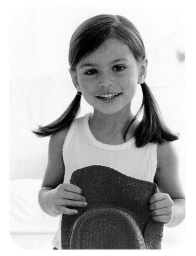
*Low pigtails*

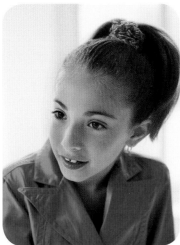
*High ponytail*

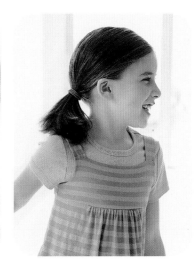
*Side ponytail*

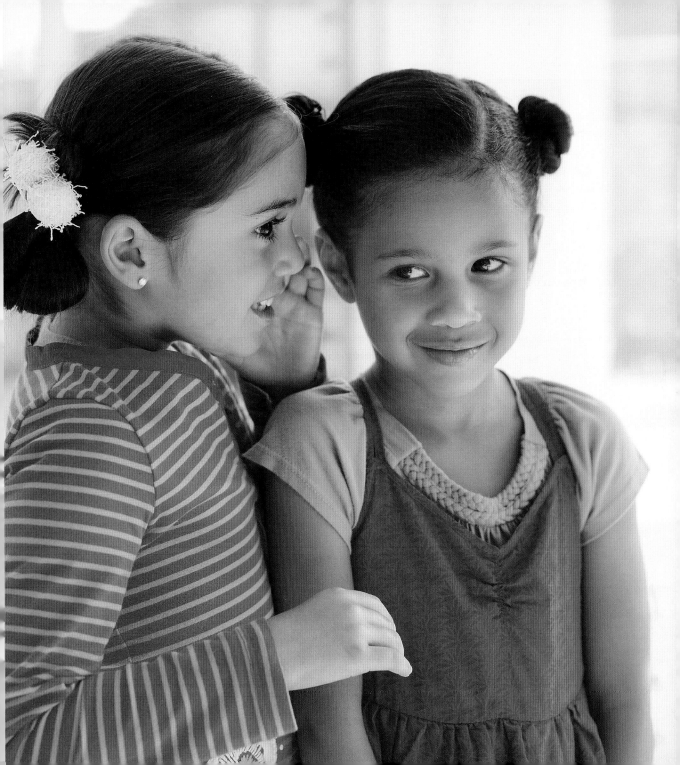

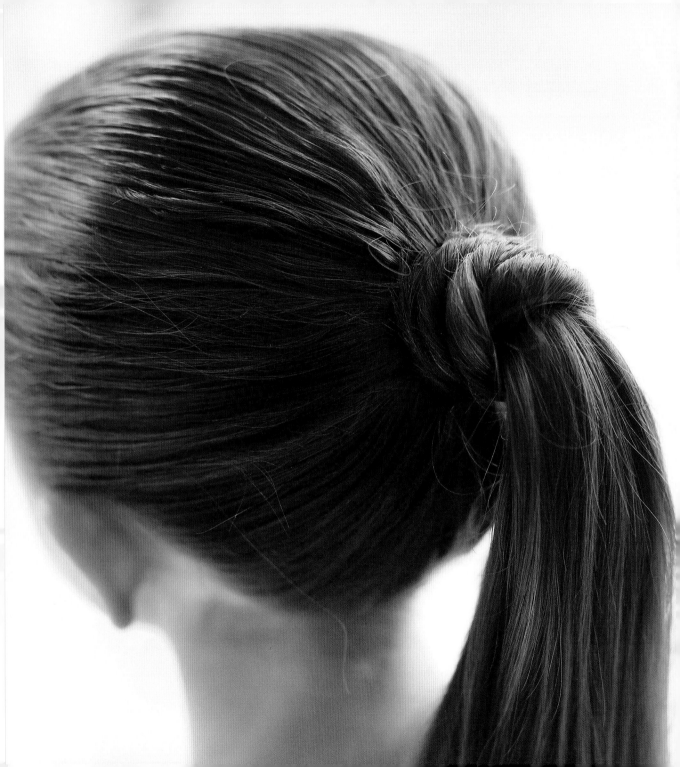

# Wrapped Ponytail

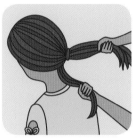

*A more polished look for a basic ponytail. This style requires longer hair.*

### What You'll Need
Comb or paddle brush
Ponytail holder
Hairpin

**Time:**
5 minutes

**Step 1:** Starting with dry hair, comb or brush the hair to smooth and detangle it.

**Step 2:** Make a high or low ponytail using a plain ponytail holder, but leave a 1-inch strand underneath the tail free from the holder (illus. 1).

**Step 3:** Wrap the 1-inch section around the base of the ponytail several times, completely covering the ponytail holder (illus. 2).

**Step 4:** Use a hairpin to secure the end of the wrapped strand to the base of the ponytail, or tuck it under the ponytail holder.

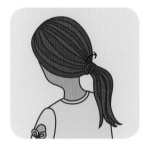

# The Flip Tail

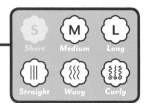

*An inside-out twist ponytail; just poke the tail through! You'll need shoulder-length or longer hair.*

### What You'll Need
Comb or paddle brush
Ponytail holder

**Time:**
5 minutes

**Step 1:** Starting with dry hair, comb or brush the hair to smooth and detangle it.

**Step 2:** Gather the hair into a low ponytail at the nape of the neck and secure it with a ponytail holder. Then push the band down slightly to leave 2 or 3 inches of hair above it.

**Step 3:** Using your pointer and middle fingers, make a "hole" in the middle of the hair above the ponytail holder. With your other hand, flip the end of the ponytail under and up through the hole.

**Step 4:** Slowly pull the ponytail through. If the ponytail sticks out from the head too much, gently pull the holder down farther to relax the style. Brush the ends of the flip tail smooth.

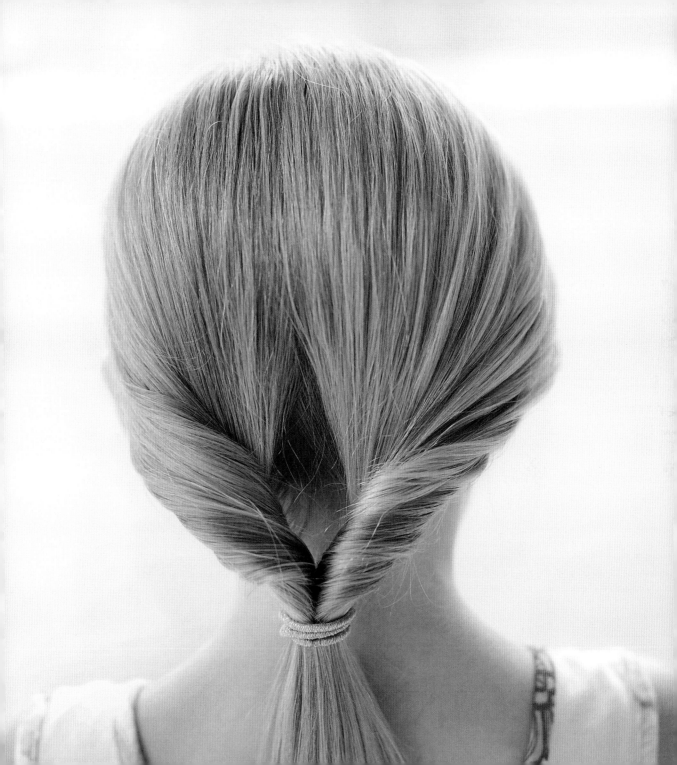

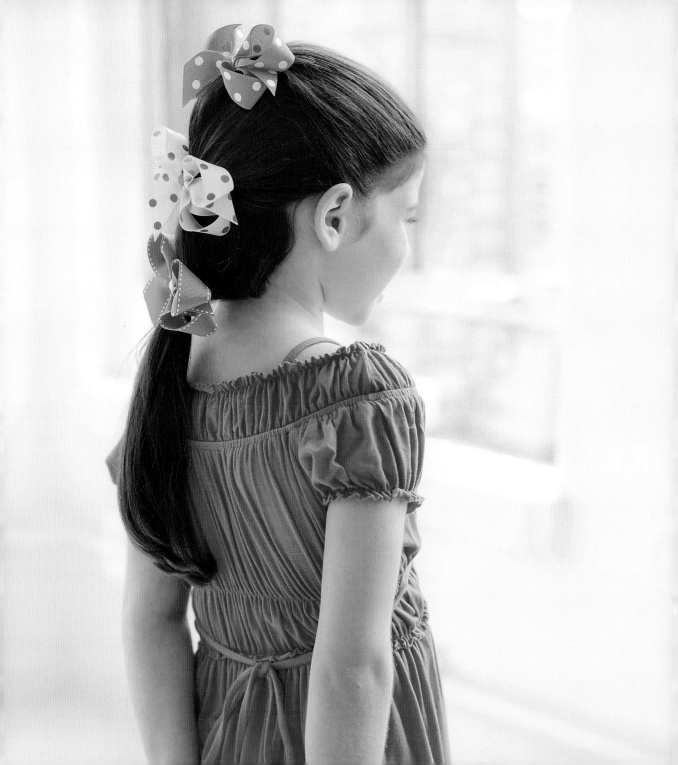

# The Bow Trio

**Short  Medium  Long**

**Straight  Wavy  Curly**

*A fancy, feminine style you can do fast.*

**What You'll Need**

Paddle brush or wide-tooth comb
Fine-tooth comb
3 small ponytail holders
3 medium to large bow clips

**Time:**
5 minutes

*Step 1:* Starting with dry hair, brush (or comb with the wide-tooth comb) the hair to smooth and detangle it.

*Step 2:* Using the fine-tooth comb, part the hair horizontally from the top of one ear to the top of the other. Comb the hair on top of the part straight back, pulling it into a ponytail that sits at midhead. Secure with a small ponytail holder (illus. 1).

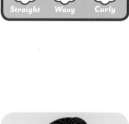

*Step 3:* Part the hair horizontally again just below the first part, at about midear. Secure with a ponytail holder just beneath the first ponytail; this is ponytail number 2 (illus. 2).

*Step 4:* Gather the remaining hair in the same way into ponytail number 3. Secure with a ponytail holder at the nape of the neck.

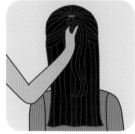

*Step 5:* Now add a pretty bow clip to cover each of the ponytail holders. You can choose the same color and pattern or three different ones.

# The Genie Ponytail

| S | M | L |
|---|---|---|
| Short | Medium | Long |
| ||| | ((( | {{{ |
| Straight | Wavy | Curly |

*This magical style for long hair can be created in the blink of an eye!*

**What You'll Need**

Comb or paddle brush
Ponytail holder
Several bobby pins
Curling iron, preheated
Hair spray

***Time:***
5–10 minutes

**Step 1:** Sweep hair back, smoothing it with a comb or paddle brush, into a high ponytail at the top of the head. Secure the ponytail with a ponytail holder. Gather a 1-inch section of hair from the lower side of the ponytail (illus. 1).

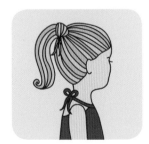

**Step 2:** Wrap the 1-inch section of hair around the base of the ponytail several times, completely covering the ponytail holder. Secure the end with bobby pins, crisscrossed for added security (illus. 2).

**Step 3:** Using the curling iron, curl the ends of the ponytail so they flip up.

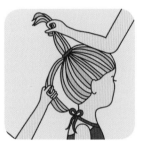

**Step 4:** Fan out the curls, then lightly mist them with hair spray.

**VARIATION**

*Add detail to this style by braiding the 1-inch section of hair before wrapping it around the base of the ponytail.*

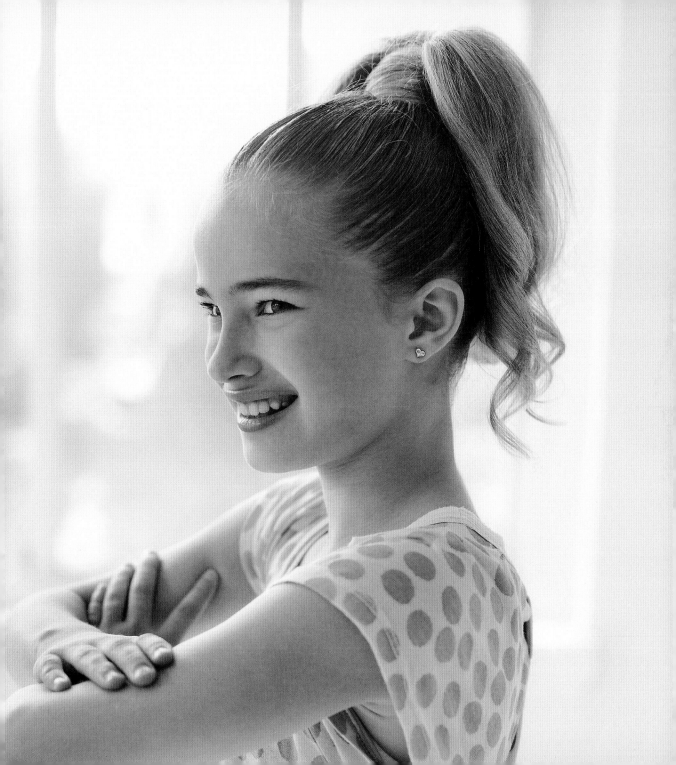

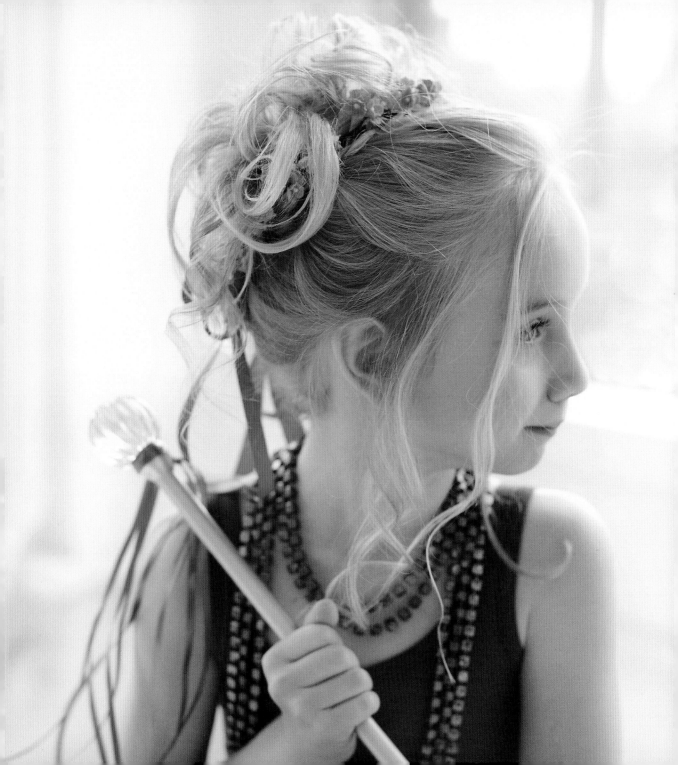

# Fairy Princess

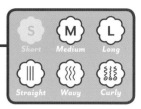

*Break out the tiaras and magic wands and practice casting enchanted spells. Have a royal tea party with pals. Whatever she does, she'll feel like she sparkles and shines in this fantasy hairstyle.*

### What You'll Need

Paddle brush or wide-tooth comb
Fine-tooth comb
Ponytail holders
Curling iron, preheated
Tiara or ribboned wreath (optional)

Hair glitter (optional)

**Time:**
15+ minutes

**Step 1:** Starting with dry hair, brush (or comb with the wide-tooth comb) it smooth and detangle it. Use the fine-tooth comb to section the hair from the top of one ear to the top of the other, over the crown of the head.

**Step 2:** Brush the hair in front of the section into a ponytail at the crown (the highest point of the head). Before securing the ponytail with a ponytail holder, use the fine-tooth comb to gently pull loose a few tendrils of hair around the face on each side. Leave these hanging for now.

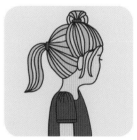

**Step 3:** Gather the remaining hair into a ponytail right below the first one, at the back middle of the head. Secure with a ponytail holder (illus. 1).

**Step 4:** Using the curling iron, wind 1- to 2-inch sections of hair from the ponytail ends around the barrel of the iron, making curls in alternating directions. Hold for no more than a few seconds or you'll damage hair (illus. 2).

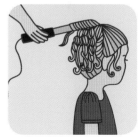

**Step 5:** Now curl the loose tendrils around the face with the iron, again holding the hair around the barrel for only a few seconds. Finish by accessorizing these royal ringlets with a tiara or a ribboned wreath. You could also spray on hair glitter for a fairy twinkle!

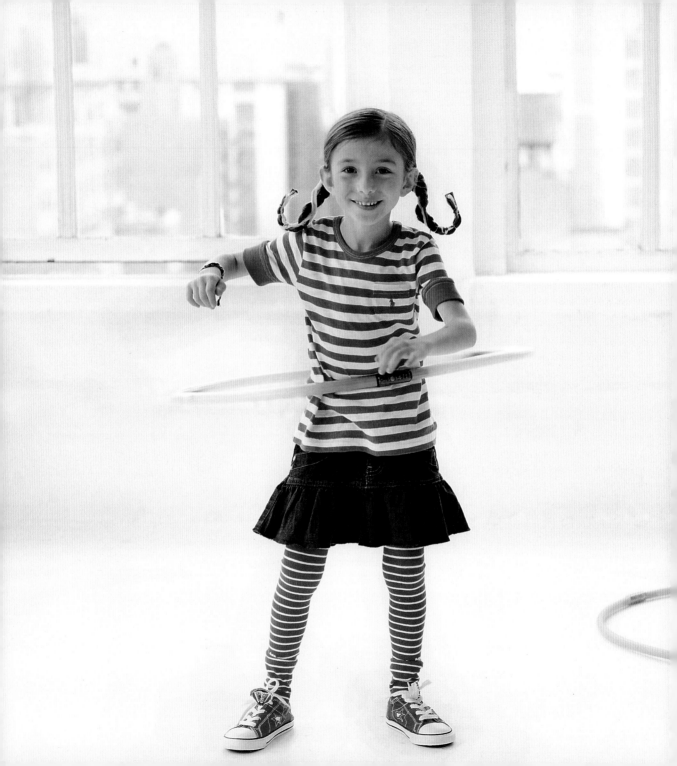

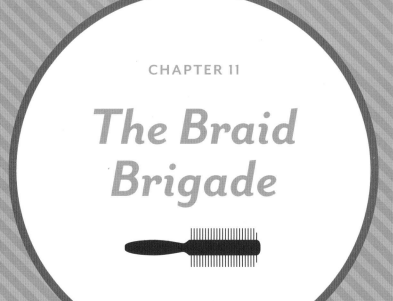

CHAPTER 11

# The Braid Brigade

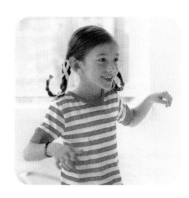

**Many parents are** afraid to braid: they think it's complicated or confusing—or they worry that their kids will never sit still long enough. Braiding does take practice, especially if you're attempting a fancy French braid or fishtail. One mom confessed that she practiced her braiding on dolls before trying it out on her three daughters! When you're ready, sit your child in front of the computer or the TV so she's distracted and not fidgeting.

While you don't need much length to create cute minibraids, fancier updo-type braids require longer hair. But no matter what type of hair you have, you can braid it! You want to work with damp hair (have a spray bottle handy) that's completely tangle-free. In general, thicker hair is easiest to braid. If your child has fine hair, it's a good idea to work in some gel to keep flyaway strands in place and the braid from slipping out. Don't forget to have ponytail holders handy to tie it all off.

Remember, too, that braids should be secure but not too tight. The tighter you pull the braids, the more you risk ripping and breaking the hair.

# The Basic Braid

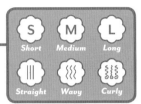

S — Short  M — Medium  L — Long

Straight  Wavy  Curly

*If you can braid, you can create so many fun styles! Here's how to make a braid that's picture-perfect every time.*

### What You'll Need

Wide-tooth comb
Fine-tooth comb
Ponytail holder

**Time:**
5 minutes

**Step 1:** Start with damp hair (either towel-dried or misted) and use the wide-tooth comb to detangle the hair.

**Step 2:** Using a fine-tooth comb, divide the hair into three equal sections as shown (illus. 1): right, left, and middle.

**Step 3:** Hold the right section in your right hand and the other two sections separately in your left. Cross the right section over the middle section and hold with your left hand (illus. 2). The original right section is now the middle section. Pull the sections away from each other to tighten the braid.

**Step 4:** Now cross the left section over the middle section (illus. 3). The original left-hand section is now the middle section. Tighten again.

**Step 5:** Continue alternating right and left sections over the middle, until you reach the end of the hair (illus. 4). Secure with a ponytail holder.

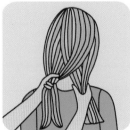

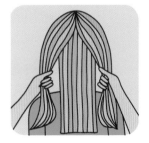

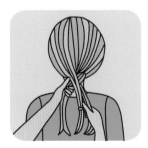

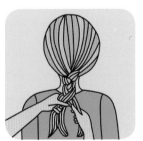

1            2            3            4

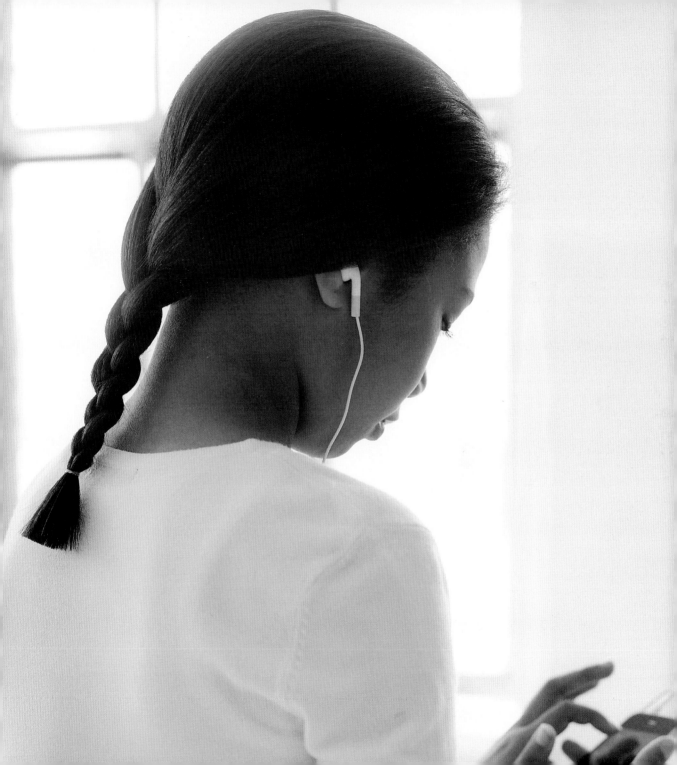

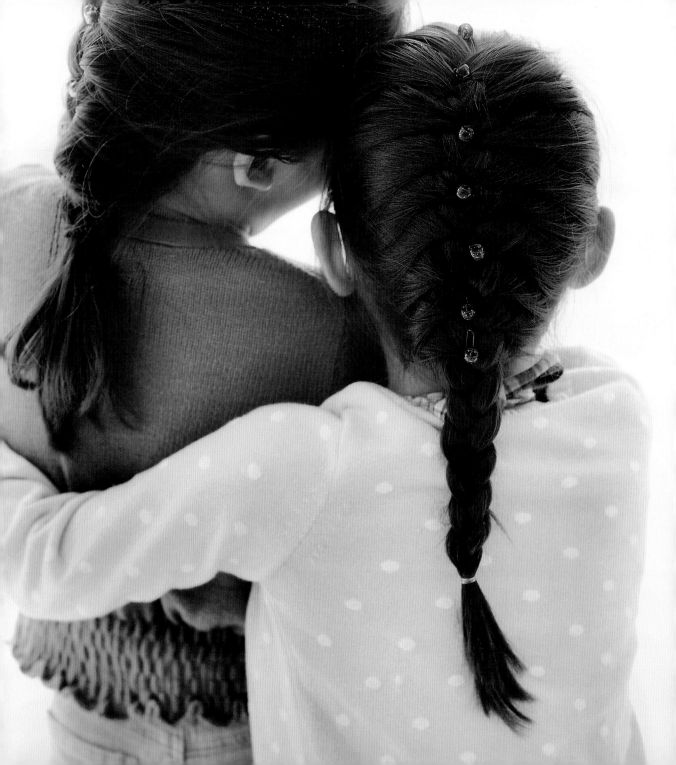

# The French Braid

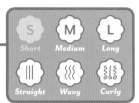

*Little girls love this ladylike look; it's an instantly dressy hairstyle for a special occasion or class pictures—or just a pretty way to pull hair out of your child's face. It looks more complicated than it is. If you can do a basic braid, you can do this as well—and the more you practice, the faster you'll get. Again, begin by either misting the hair or lightly gelling it, and make sure it's totally tangle-free.*

## What You'll Need
Wide-tooth comb
Fine-tooth comb
Ponytail holder
Hair gel (optional)

**Time:**
10–15 minutes

**Step 1:** Start with damp hair (either towel-dried or misted) and use the wide-tooth comb to detangle the hair. Measure a section of hair from the front of the head that is approximately the width of the temples. Smooth it straight back with no part, and with a fine-tooth comb, divide it into three sections (illus. 1).

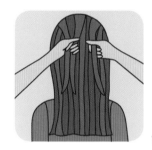

**Step 2:** Cross the left section over the center section, then cross the right section over the center section. Pull the sections away from each other to tighten the braid. (See The Basic Braid on page 140.)

**Step 3:** Beginning on the right side, use a finger (pinky or pointer works best) to gather a small strand (about 1 inch wide) of loose hair next to the right section (illus. 2). Join this hair into the right section.

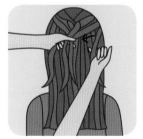

**Step 4:** Now cross this right section over the middle section, as if you're doing a basic braid. Pull the sections taut.

**Step 5:** In the same way, take a small strand of hair next to the left section and join it into the left section. Now cross the left section over the middle one (illus. 3). Pull the sections taut.

**Step 6:** Continue adding small strands of hair into the right and left sections, leaving no hair hanging free, as you braid down to the nape of the neck (illus. 4). Now divide the remaining hair at the neck into two sections (right and left) and join them into the right and left sections of the braid.

**Step 7:** Finish with a basic braid, and secure with a ponytail holder (illus. 5). Use a pea-sized amount of hair gel, rubbed between your palms, to smooth any stray strands.

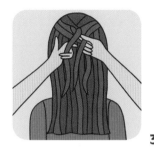

3

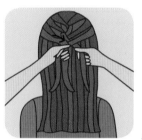

4

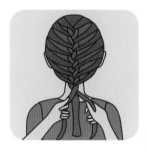

5

# The Heart Braid

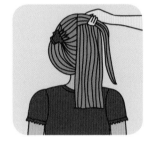

This is a gorgeous, unique style that requires an experienced braider!

## What You'll Need

Wide-tooth comb
Fine-tooth comb
Hair clip
Ponytail holders

**Time:**
15 minutes

**Step 1:** Starting with damp hair (either towel-dried or misted), use a wide-tooth comb to detangle the hair. Then, using a fine-tooth comb, part the hair down the middle of the head. Clip one side up right above the ear.

**Step 2:** On the other side of the part, use the fine comb to gather a thin section of hair from the crown. This section should measure about 2 inches from the hairline to the top of the head (illus. 1).

**1**

**Step 3:** Divide this section into three, and begin a French braid (see page 143) starting at the crown and curving toward the temple, then toward the back of the head, like the top lobe of a heart. You will be lifting hair into the braid only from this side of the part. Leave no loose hair in front of the ear (illus. 2).

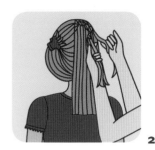

2

**Step 4:** When you reach the center part at the back of the head, secure the braid with a ponytail holder. If the hair is very long, end the braid about midear; the ends will hang down the back (illus. 3).

**Step 5:** Unclip the hair on the other side of the part and repeat the process. Secure with a ponytail holder.

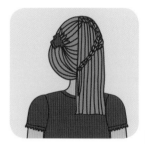

3

**Step 6:** Join the two ends of the braids together in the back with a ponytail holder to form the bottom point of the heart (illus. 4).

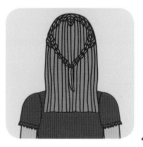

4

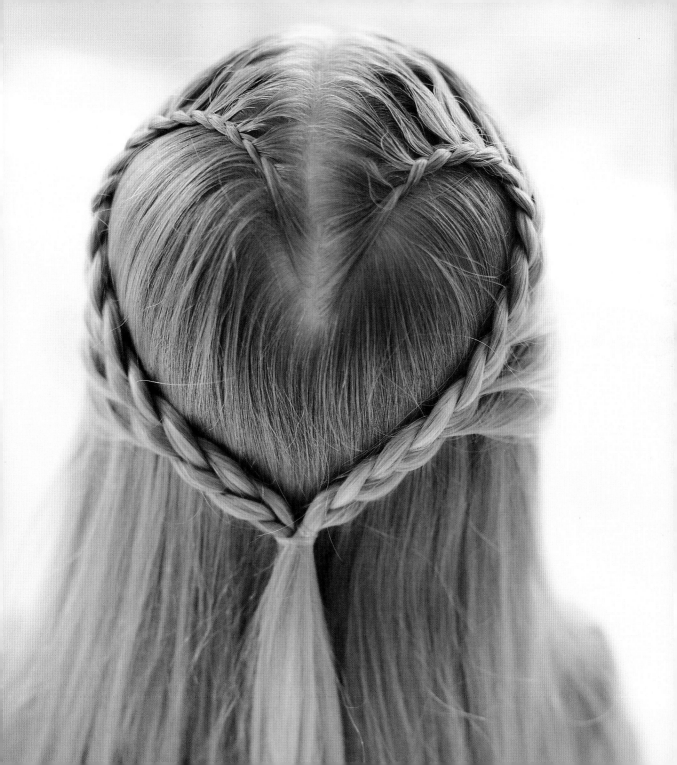

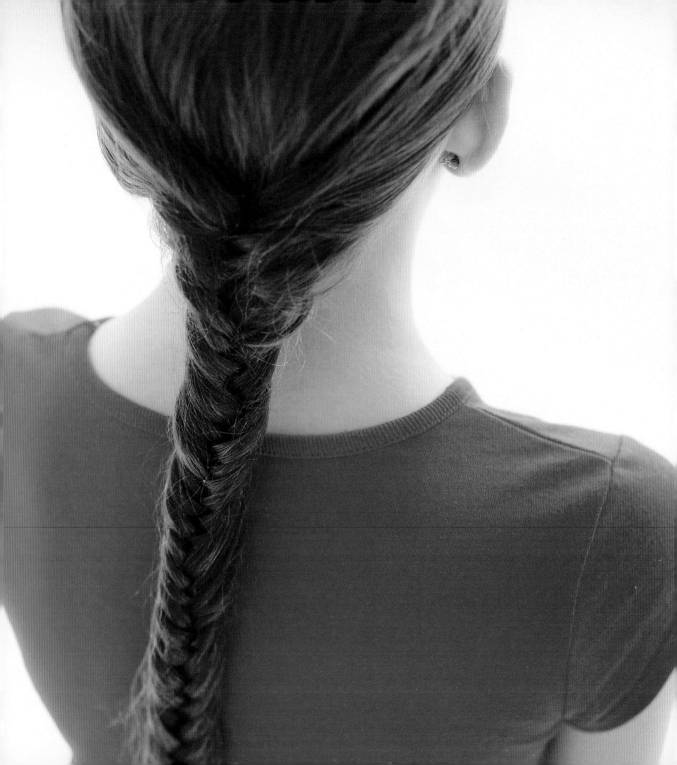

# The Fishtail Braid

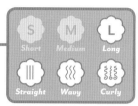

*Also called the herringbone, this braid looks impressively intricate, especially on long hair. Don't be intimidated; once you understand the hand placement, it practically braids itself.*

**What You'll Need**

Wide-tooth comb
Ponytail holders

**Time:**

15 minutes

**Step 1:** Start with damp hair (either towel-dried or misted) and use the wide-tooth comb to detangle the hair.

**Step 2:** Divide the hair into two equal sections at the nape of the neck. If you're a beginner, try starting with a ponytail, placing the elastic at the nape of the neck. Divide the ponytail into two equal sections, right and left (illus. 1).

**Step 3:** Hold the right section with your right hand. Using your left hand, gather a skinny (about ⅛ inch wide) strand of hair from the outside of the left section and cross it over to the inside of the right section (illus. 2), now holding that section with your right hand. You should now have two sections again; the left (missing that strand of hair), and the right with the strand you just incorporated. Pull the braid taut.

**Step 4:** Now hold the left section in your left hand. Use your right hand to pick up a skinny strand of hair from the outside of the right section and cross it over to the inside of the left section, now holding that section with your left hand. Again, you're left with two sections (illus. 3). Pull taut.

**Step 5:** Continue picking up small sections from the outside of one section and joining them to the inside of the other. Once you get into a groove, it's easy! When you reach the end, secure the braid with a ponytail holder.

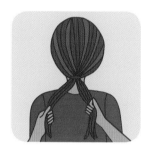

2

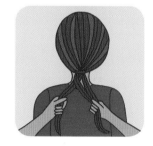

3

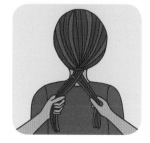

# Minibraids

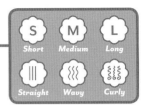

S — Short  M — Medium  L — Long

Straight  Wavy  Curly

*These whimsical braids are playful and fun to accessorize. An added plus:*
*They work for any hair length—short, long, or in-between.*

### What You'll Need

Wide-tooth comb
Fine-tooth comb
Ponytail holders
Small hair clips

**Time:**
10 minutes

**Step 1:** Start with damp hair (either towel-dried or misted) and use the wide-tooth comb to detangle the hair. Use the fine-tooth comb to part the hair to one side.

**Step 2:** On the side of the part with more hair, gather a section of hair along the part, extending approximately 2 inches back from the hairline (illus. 1).

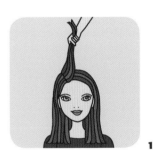

1

**Step 3:** Braid that section on a diagonal, directed toward the back of the head. Secure with a ponytail holder (illus. 2).

**Step 4:** Flip the braid over to the other side of the part so it's out of your way. Using the fine-tooth comb, gather a second section of hair farther away from the part, starting about 1½ inches from the hairline and extending approximately 3½ inches back from the hairline (illus. 3). Again, braid on the diagonal and secure with a ponytail holder.

2

**Step 5:** Flip the second braid to the other side of the part. Now gather a third section of hair next to the second braid and slightly farther up the part. Braid on the diagonal and secure with a ponytail holder.

**Step 6:** Put cute clips at the top of each braid to accessorize and to keep the braids from falling in the child's face.

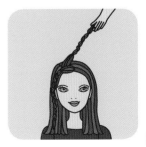

3

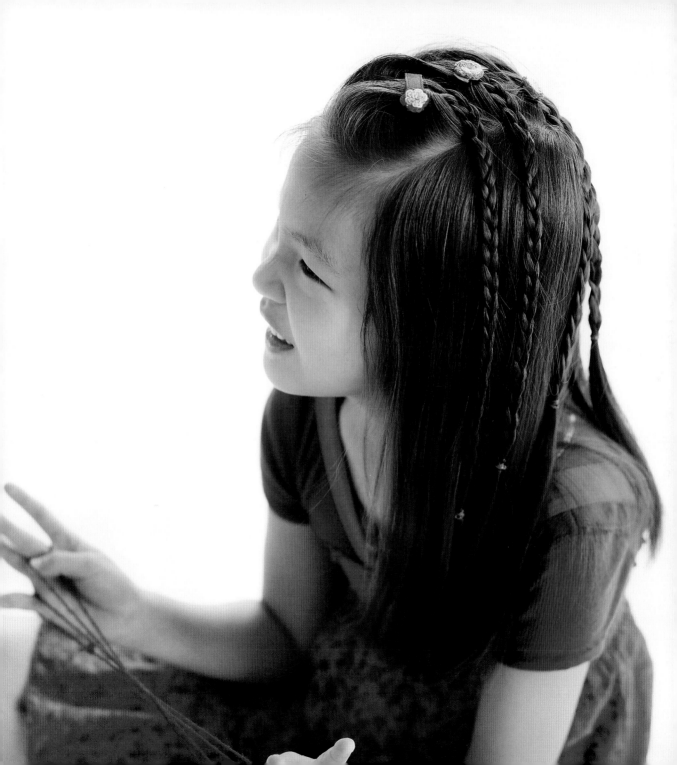

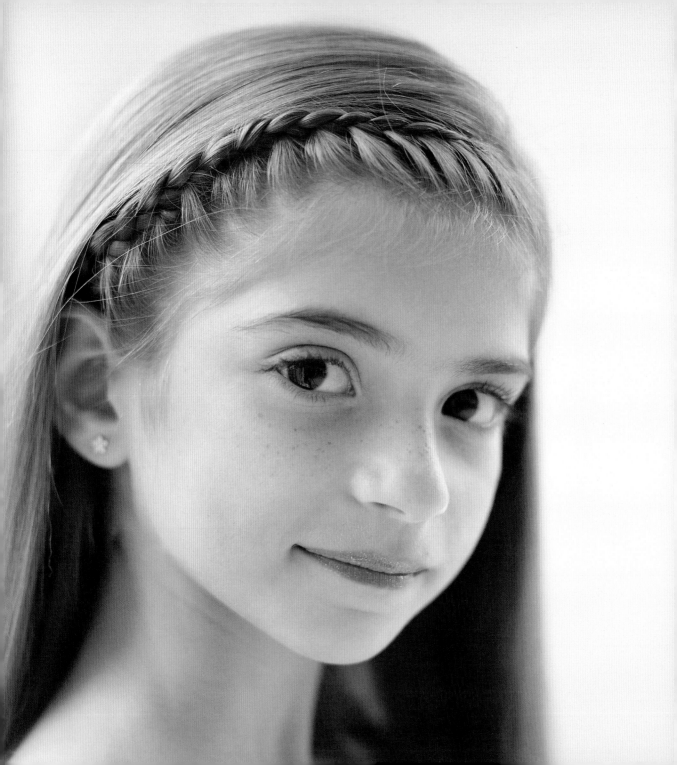

# The French Braid Headband

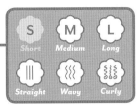

*Besides being a great way to keep hair off the face, this braided band makes its own accessory. Girls can wear it with their hair hanging down in back, or with a ponytail, bun, or larger braid.*

### What You'll Need

Wide-tooth comb

Fine-tooth comb

Ponytail holders

Jaw clip

Bobby pins

***Time:***

10–15 minutes

**Step 1:** Start with damp hair (either towel-dried or misted) and use a wide-tooth comb to detangle the hair.

**Step 2:** Use a fine-tooth comb to draw a horizontal line across the crown from the top of one ear to the top of the other ear. From the line, comb the hair forward to the face. Pull the hair in back of the line into a ponytail holder or jaw clip so it stays out of your way.

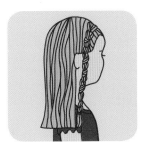

**Step 3:** Choose which ear you want the braid to start from. Tilt the head so the ear you've chosen is facing up toward the ceiling. With your child's ear tilted up, begin making the braided headband using the hair in front of the part. French-braid (see page 143) tightly across the crown and down to the other side, gathering small (¼- to ½-inch) sections from above the part (illus.).

**Step 4:** Once you've reached the other ear, secure the braid with a ponytail holder. If you like, tuck it behind the ear and pin it in place with a few bobby pins. Remove the ponytail holder or jaw clip used in Step 2 and style as you like.

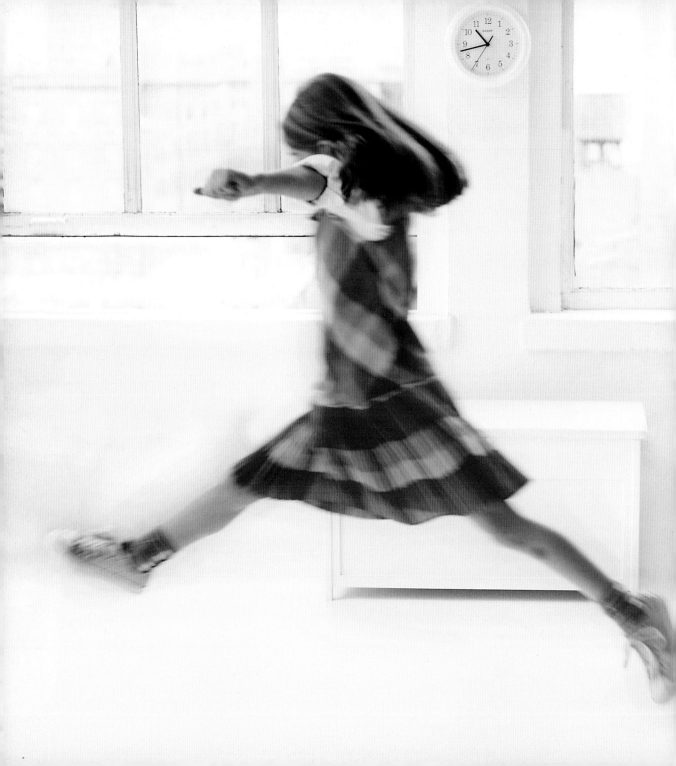

# CHAPTER 12

# Five Under-5-Minute Styles

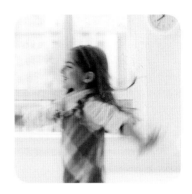

*It's 8:15 A.M.,* and you're breathlessly racing to get your kid out the door to school. You hate the idea of sending her off looking like she fell out of bed (even if she did). Luckily, these styles can be done with lightning speed (under five minutes—promise!) and are perfect for those mornings when time is not on your side. Try to keep all hair gear in one place: brushes, combs, and spray-in conditioner can sit on a dresser top or on a shelf in the bathroom. It will make it that much easier to grab and go.

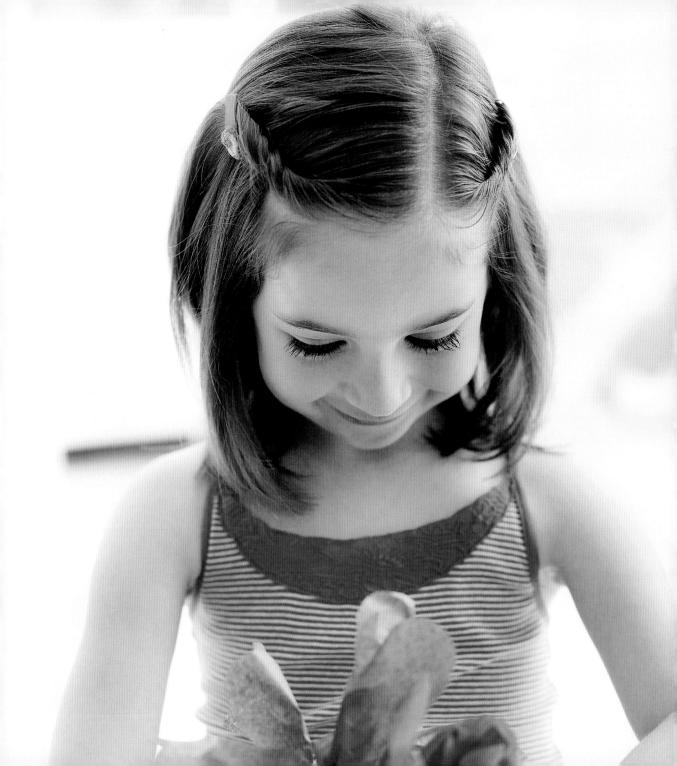

# The Double Twist

*This is a dainty look for little ones. You can use matching barrettes or ones that cutely clash.*

S Short   M Medium   L Long

Straight   Wavy   Curly

## What You'll Need

Brush or wide-tooth comb
Fine-tooth comb

Small barrettes or hair clips
Bobby pins (optional)

**Step 1:** Starting with dry or damp hair, use the brush or wide-tooth comb to remove tangles. Using the fine-tooth comb, part hair either in the middle or to one side.

**Step 2:** Gather a small section of hair, approximately an inch wide, from one side of the part at the front of the head. Tightly twist the section (but not so tight that it hurts!) toward the part, so the twist "opens" upward rather than downward. Keep the twist close to the scalp, working in more hair as you go, and ending the twist at the crown of the head. Secure with a pretty clip at the crown.

**Step 3:** Repeat on the other side of the part. If hair is fine—and the barrette might slide off—you may want to secure the twists with bobby pins before adding the clip.

# The Basic Bun

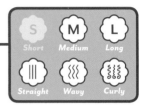

*This simple way of scooping hair up always makes girls feel grown-up. Don't make the bun too tight or severe; a softer style is not only prettier, but also more comfy.*

### What You'll Need

Wide-tooth comb

Ponytail holder

Several bobby pins

Hair spray

**Step 1:** Starting with damp hair, comb through to smooth and remove tangles.

**Step 2:** Gather hair in a loose ponytail. Position the ponytail where you want the bun to be on the head: low at the nape, middle of the head, or high on the crown. Secure with a ponytail holder.

**Step 3:** Twist the ponytail into a tight rope, coiling it around itself at the base (illus. 1).

**Step 4:** Tuck the ends of the coil into the ponytail holder at the base (illus. 2). Then secure the bun by pushing bobby pins into the hair at the bun's base on all sides. The thicker the hair, the more pins you'll need. Lightly spritz the bun with hair spray to lock in the style.

### VARIATION

*The Tropical Twist: Make the bun to one side of the head, positioning the coil just behind the ear. Decorate the bun with fresh or faux flowers or leaves.*

*The Choppy Bun: Poke a pair of painted chopsticks through the bun, crisscrossing them in the middle.*

*The Undone Bun: Instead of coiling hair tightly, create a loosely twisted bun, secure with a ponytail holder, and leave the ends untucked and unpinned. You can also pull a few tendrils loose on the sides.*

*The Braided Bun: Make a braided ponytail, tying it off with a ponytail holder before you make the coil of the bun.*

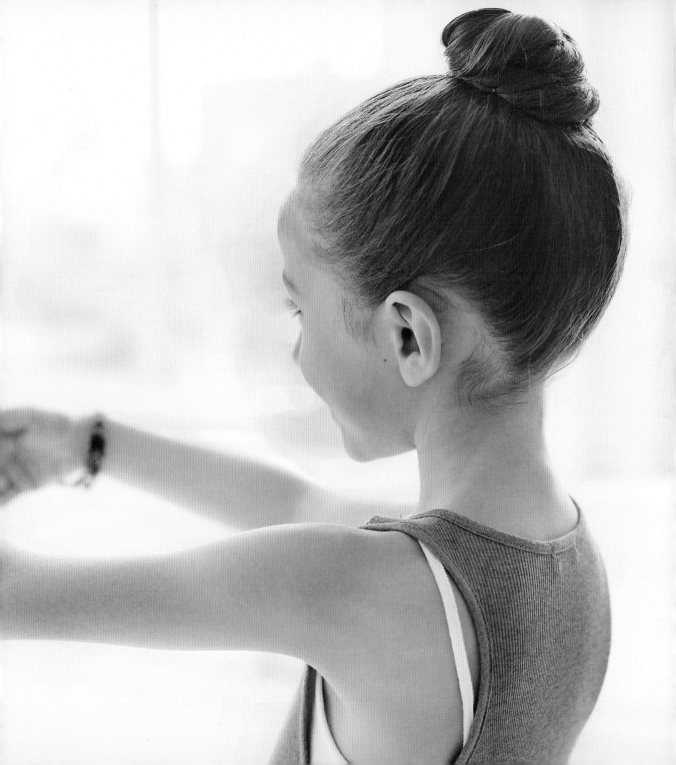

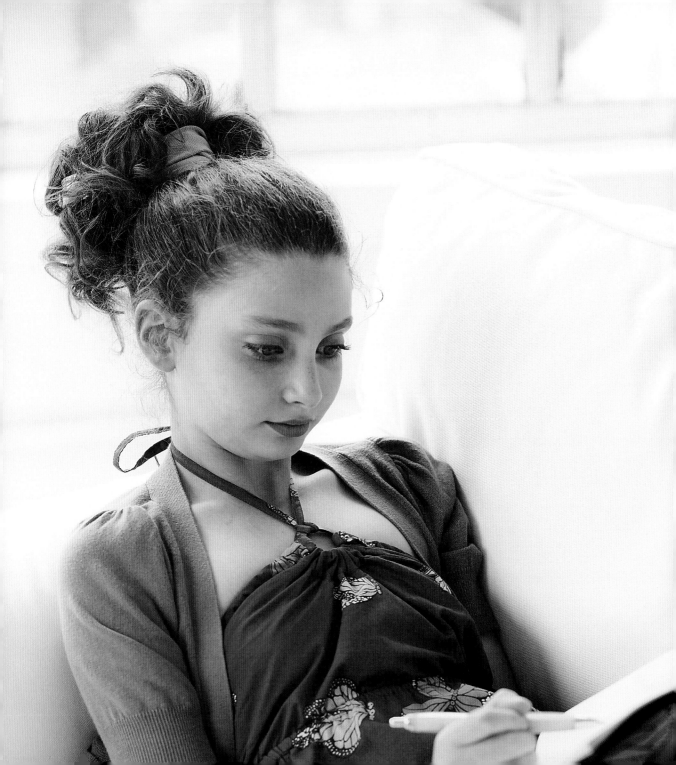

# The Carefree Ponytail

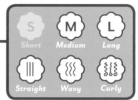

*Here's a casual, carefree style you can't do wrong! Don't fuss too much with it; you want the ends to appear a bit unkempt while the top of the head is smooth.*

## What You'll Need

Brush or wide-tooth comb          Mousse or gel
Ponytail holder or scrunchie

**Step 1:** Starting with dry or damp hair, brush or comb the hair back at the crown and sides.

**Step 2:** Grasp the hair with both hands, and gather it into a loose ponytail at the back of the head. The easiest position is about midhead, but you can make it higher or lower, or even position the ponytail to the side. Secure with a ponytail holder or scrunchie.

**Step 3:** Rub a dime-sized amount of mousse or gel between your hands and run them through the ponytail. Fluff and scrunch the hair to create a "messy" cascade.

# The Wispy Loop

*Up, up, and away! This style sweeps hair off the face and neck in a flash.*

### What You'll Need
Brush or wide-tooth comb          Large butterfly clip

**Step 1:** Starting with dry hair, brush or comb hair to detangle. Part it where you choose, or smooth hair straight back.

**Step 2:** Gather the hair in the center of the head as if you were making a ponytail. Twist the hair up and around loosely (more looped than coiled) in an elongated bun shape, leaving a few short wispy ends sticking out at top or bottom.

**Step 3:** Secure with the clip at the center of the twist to hold the style in place.

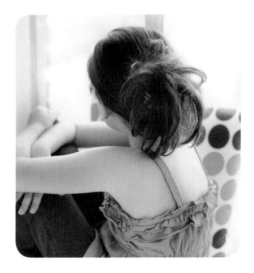

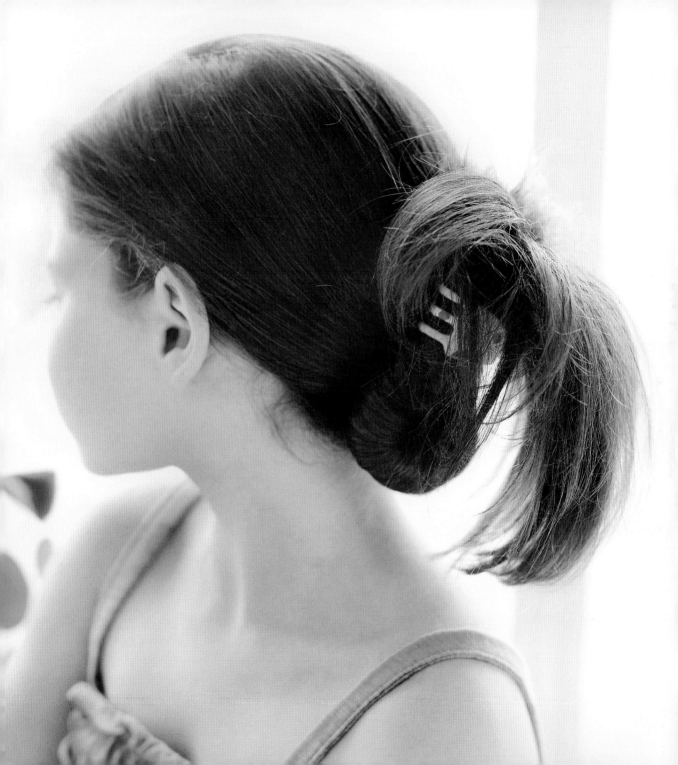

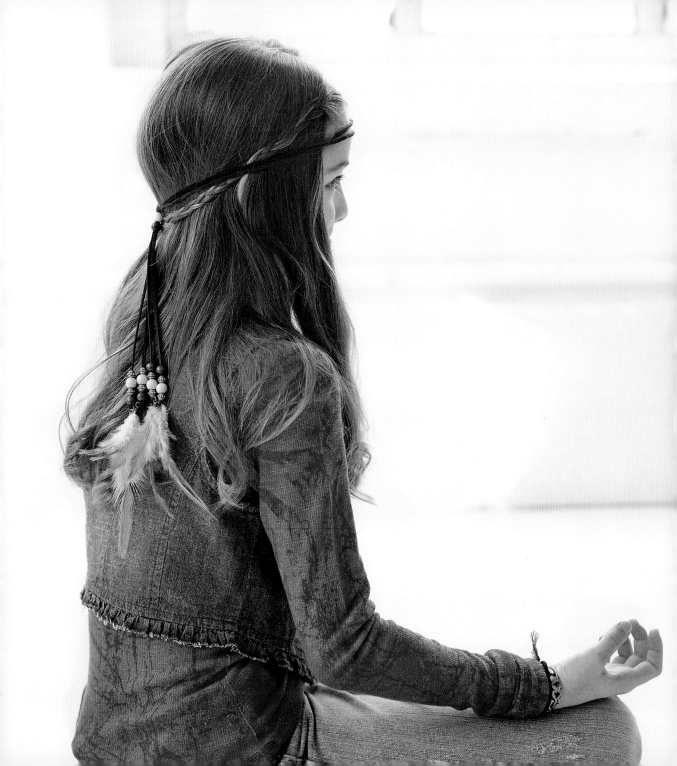

# The Hippie Chick

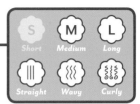

*There's nothing fussy or frilly about this all-natural flower child. Heavily accessorized with feathers, flowers, or beads, this can be a fantasy hairstyle; with no extras, it's an easy look for everyday wear. The hair should be long enough to create braids that can be joined behind the head. Any accessories can be pushed into the braid, or tucked in at the hairline or beneath the ponytail holder.*

### What You'll Need

Brush or wide-tooth comb

Spray bottle of water

Fine-tooth comb

Small ponytail holders

**Step 1:** Starting with dry hair, brush or comb the hair to smooth and detangle it. Lightly mist it with water so it is slightly damp. Using the fine-tooth comb, part hair in the center.

**Step 2:** On one side of the part near the hairline, pick up a 1-inch section of hair and braid it (see illus.). Secure with a small ponytail holder.

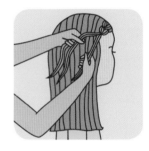

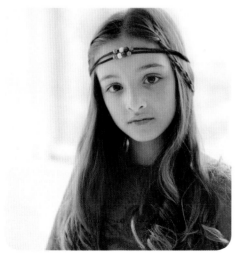

**Step 3:** Repeat on the other side of the part, to create a second braid. Join the ends of the two braids together with a small ponytail holder at the back of the head. Leave the remaining hair loose, flowing, and natural.

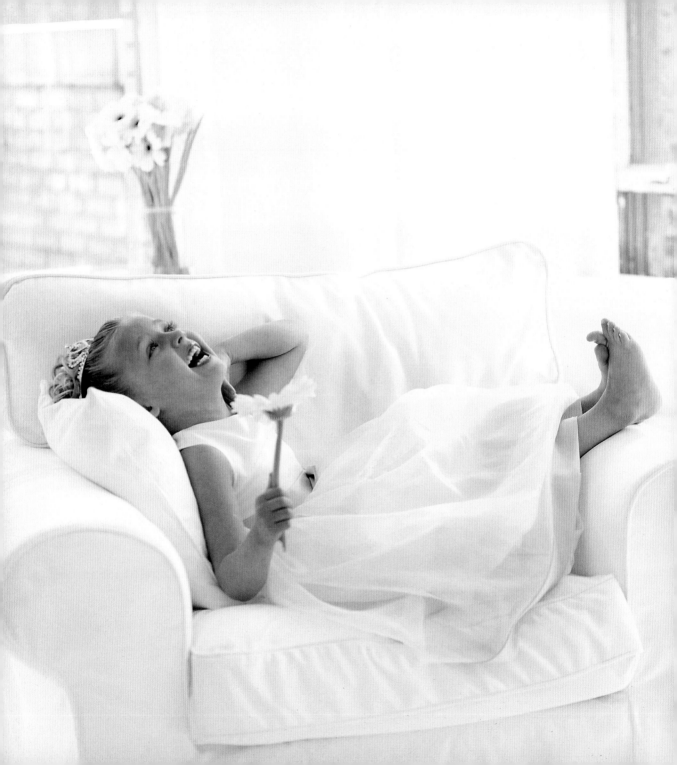

# CHAPTER 13

# Special Occasion Styles

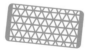

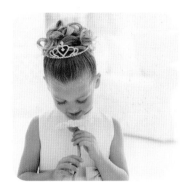

*Formal events—like* weddings, bat mitzvahs, first
communions, and holiday parties—call for special styles that are
a bit more fancy than everyday looks. Just as you'd spend time
picking out the perfect dress and shoes, you should also spend
time selecting a hairstyle that suits the occasion and your child.
Little girls love updos and accessorizing hair; usually, anything that
projects princess or ballerina is bound to be a hit. Older girls like
sophisticated styles that mimic mom . . . or Hollywood glamour.
Play dress-up before the Big Day: have your child get decked out
in her outfit and practice the style on her to see if you can do it and
how long it lasts.

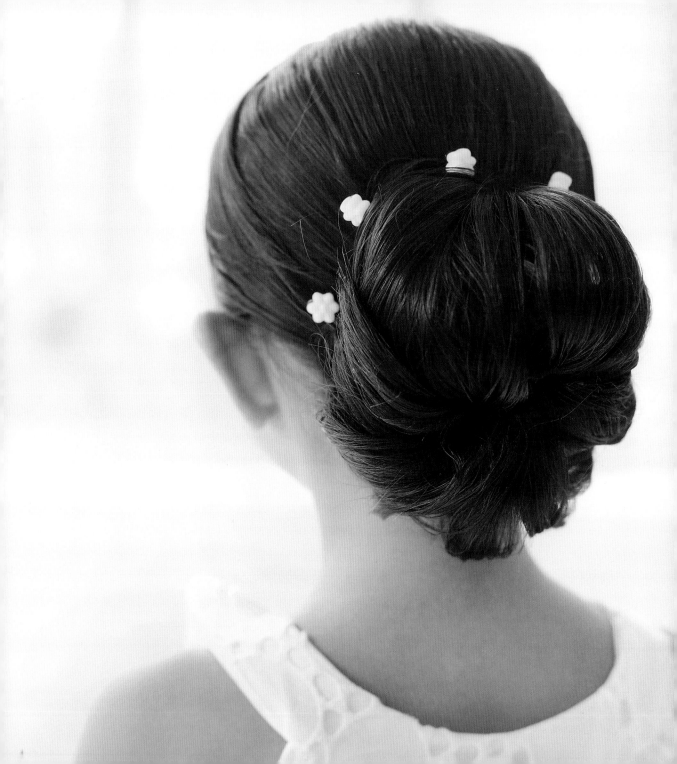

# The Ballerina Chignon

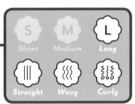

This graceful look is often thought of as a classic ballerina style and looks lovely when worn with a full skirt that twirls. The chignon dates back to ancient Greece, where women frequently wore it adorned with gold and ivory ornamentation. The style has been popular throughout time because of its association with elegance and the ease with which it can be created. You can make this even fancier by placing small pearl or sparkly beads on hairpins and planting them along the top of the chignon.

**What You'll Need**

Comb or paddle brush
Fine-tooth comb
Ponytail holders
Several hairpins

Sparkly or pearl beads (optional)

**Time:**
5–10 minutes

**Step 1:** Starting with dry hair, comb or brush the hair to smooth and detangle it. Let hair fall where it naturally parts.

**Step 2:** Using a fine-tooth comb, section top front portion of hair horizontally, from the top of one ear to the top of the other ear (illus. 1). Pull the lower section of hair back into a ponytail and secure with a ponytail holder.

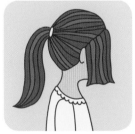

**Step 3:** Comb the front section straight back neatly and use hairpins to pin the hair into the ponytail base (illus. 2). This will make the sides of the style neat and sleek.

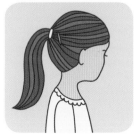

**Step 4:** Split the ponytail in half horizontally. Comb the top section up and roll it up into a loop (illus. 3). Using 2 or 3 hairpins (depending on the thickness of the hair), pin the ends to the base of the ponytail.

**Step 5:** Comb the lower section of hair down. Rolling it under, make a loop. Use hairpins to pin the ends to the base of the ponytail.

**Step 6:** Using several hairpins, stretch out the loops of hair all around the ponytail base, so the loops each form a semicircle—one on the top and one on the bottom (illus. 4). If you wish, add small sparkly or pearl beads to hairpins and crown the top of the chignon.

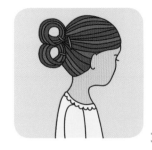

3

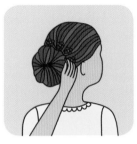

4

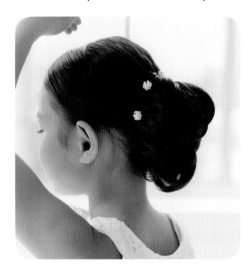

# The Ponytail Veil

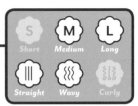

Also called the spider's web, this style joins mini-ponytails together down the back of the head in a spectacular woven pattern. Accessorize this style by pinning in small beads or attaching mini–butterfly clips at each of the ponytail holders. Or simply use different-colored bands to make this web more whimsical! Note: If hair is short or has shorter layers, do fewer links or keep them closer together (about 1 inch between the elastics instead of 2).

## What You'll Need

Wide-tooth comb or paddle brush
Spray bottle of water
Fine-tooth comb
Several ponytail holders

Beads, hairpins, mini–butterfly clips
   to accessorize (optional)

**Time:**
15+ minutes

**Step 1:** Starting with dry hair, comb or brush the hair to smooth and detangle it. Mist with the spray bottle to make the hair damp but not wet. Then comb it straight back with no part.

**Step 2:** Lift a small 1-inch section of hair (about the distance between the eyebrows) at the crown (the topmost part of the head) and make it into a small ponytail at the top of the head. Secure with a ponytail holder.

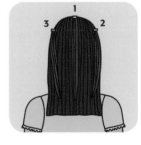

**Step 3:** Using the fine-tooth comb, gather a 1-inch section from each side of the crown and make two more ponytails in the back, securing them with ponytail holders about 1 inch below the center ponytail. Now you have 3 ponytails (illus. 1).

**Step 4:** Split ponytail #1 in two. Then split ponytail #2 in two. Join the right half of ponytail #1 to the left half of ponytail #2 and secure them with a ponytail holder about 2 inches below ponytail #2's holder. This makes ponytail #4 (illus. 2).

**Step 5:** Now split ponytail #3 in two and join its right side to the left half of ponytail #1. Secure with a ponytail holder about 2 inches below ponytail #3's holder. This makes ponytail #5 (illus. 2).

**Step 6:** Split ponytail #4 in two. Join the right half of ponytail #2 to the right half of ponytail #4, securing with a ponytail holder about 2 inches below ponytail #4's holder. This makes ponytail #6 (illus. 3).

**Step 7:** Split ponytail #5 in two. Now join the left half of ponytail #3 to the left half of ponytail #5, securing with a ponytail holder about 2 inches below ponytail #5's holder. This makes ponytail #7 (illus. 3).

**Step 8:** Now join the left half of ponytail #4 with the right half of ponytail #5. Secure with a ponytail holder to make ponytail #8.

**Step 9:** Now gather a thin 1-inch section of hair from behind each ear and combine with all of ponytail #6 on the right and all of ponytail #7 on the left. Secure each with a ponytail holder to make ponytails #9 and #10.

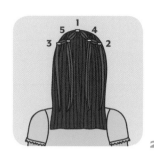

2

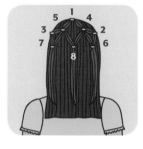

3

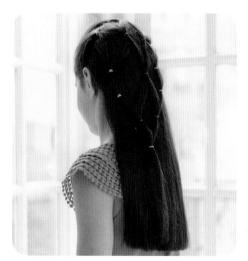

**Step 10:** Depending on hair length, you can continue creating a web of ponytails down the back. When you're done, gather all the ponytail ends together and secure with a ponytail holder.

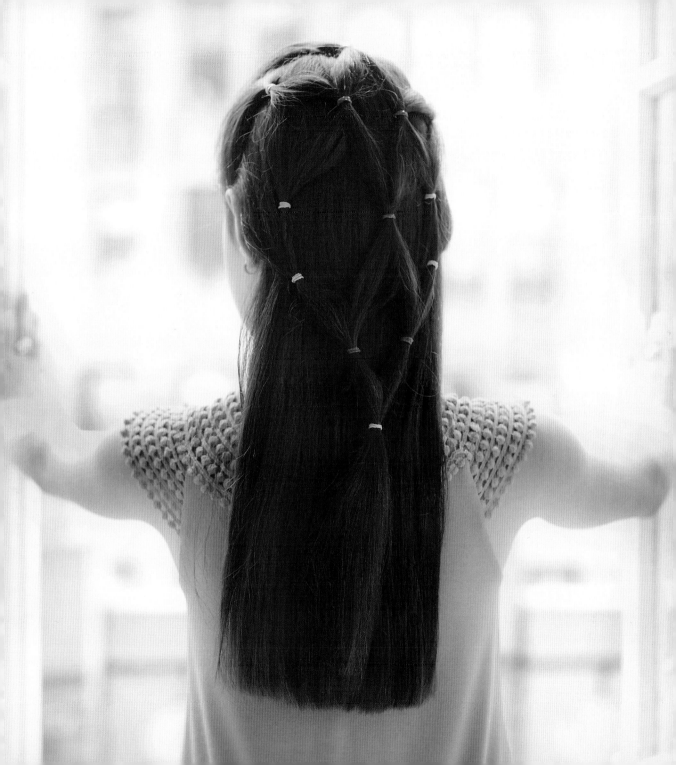

# The Wraparound

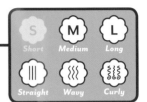

*This star-inspired style—often seen on the red carpet—works for medium to long hair, both straight and curly.*

## What You'll Need

Spray bottle of water

Fine-tooth comb

Ponytail holders

Curling iron, preheated

Several hairpins

***Time:***

10–15 minutes

**Step 1:** Start with dry hair. Mist the hair with the spray bottle to make it damp but not wet.

**Step 2:** Using a fine-tooth comb, part the hair to one side and, on the side with more hair, gather a 3-inch section of hair along the part, starting at the forehead. Make a French braid (see page 143), pulling in hair only from the side of the part the braid is on. The braid should go in the same direction as the part, toward the back of the head (illus. 1). Braid through to the ends, and secure with a ponytail holder.

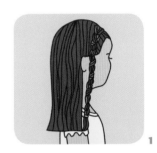

**Step 3:** Make a ponytail at the nape of the neck with the remaining hair. Secure with a ponytail holder.

**Step 4:** Split the ponytail into several 1-inch sections and curl each one downward with a curling iron. Use hairpins to pin these tendrils to the base of the ponytail in alternating directions (illus. 2). The look is messy.

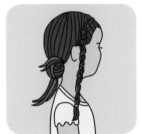

**Step 5:** Once you have your messy bun, wind the braid around the base of the bun and pin the end underneath (illus. 3). If the hair is too short to allow you to wind the braid, you can tuck it into the side of the bun.

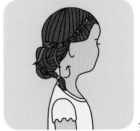

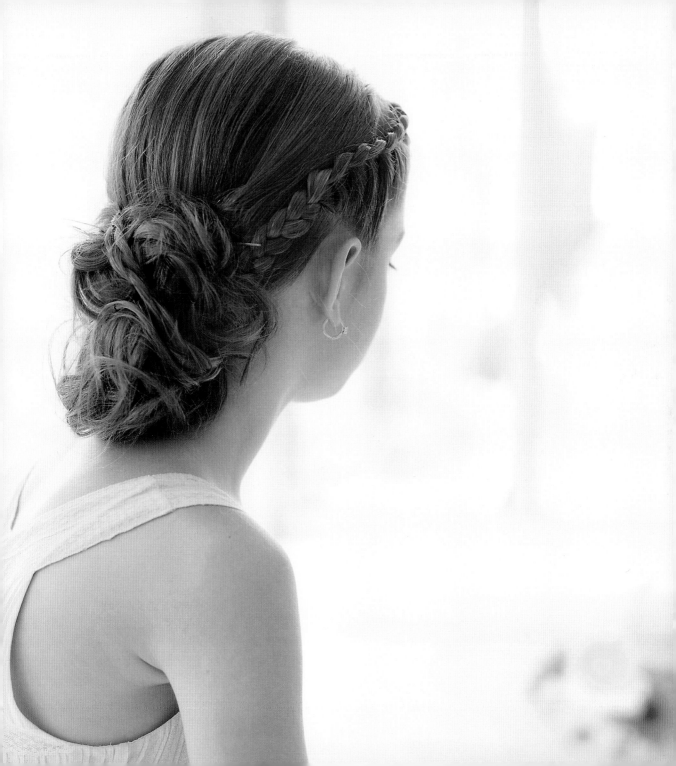

# The French Twist

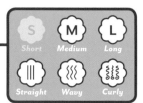

The French twist became popular during the Victorian era of the nineteenth century in contrast to the elaborate styles and curls that were popular during the preceding Georgian era. Simple hairstyles emphasizing natural beauty were the trend during the Victorian era, and they still look stylish today.

### What You'll Need

Comb or paddle brush
Hair gel or light styling cream
Several bobby pins

**Time:**
10 minutes

**Step 1:** Starting with dry hair, comb or brush the hair to smooth and detangle it. Rub a pea-sized amount of gel between your palms and smooth the top and sides back. Gather the hair as if you were going to make a ponytail at midhead (illus. 1).

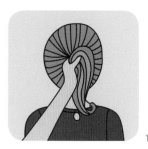

**Step 2:** Begin twisting the hair in a clockwise direction, pulling it upward at the same time. The ends should be pointing up as you twist tightly (illus. 2). Tuck the coil tightly against the head with your other hand as you twist. Stop when you have a few pointy ends sticking up at the top of the coil.

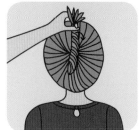

**Step 3:** Place bobby pins all along the length of the coil to attach it to the head (illus. 3). You can fan the ends or tuck and pin them under for an even sleeker style.

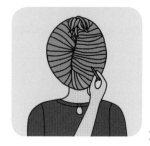

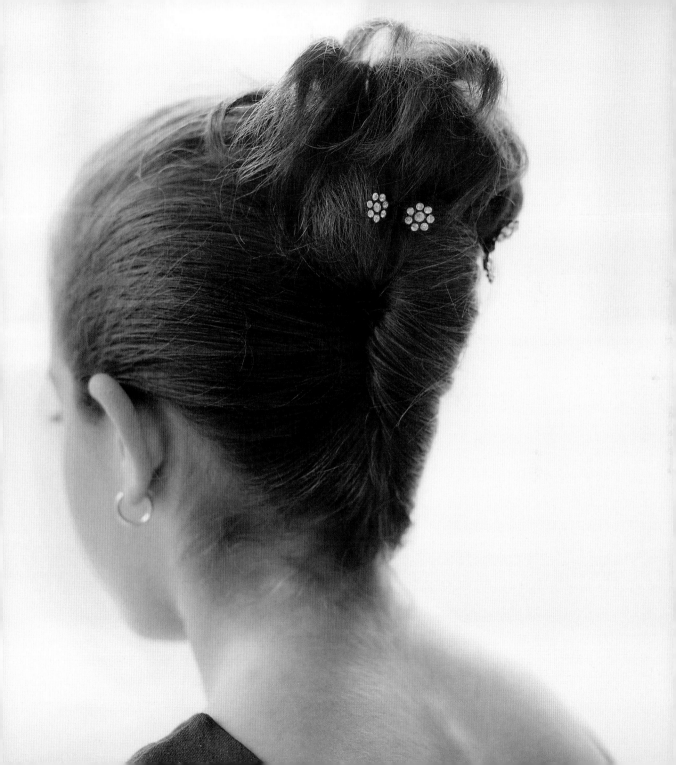

## *Picture-Perfect Hair*

Now that you know how to create so many gorgeous styles for your child, try them out every day—or on special occasions. We bet this year's class picture will be the best one yet! Here's how to get hair camera-ready for class photos.

- Get hair cut two weeks before, not the day before . . . just in case! The hair will look more natural and you'll have a little time to fix it (and let it grow in a bit) if you're not completely happy with the haircut.

- Shampoo the night before, not the morning of (unless your child usually shampoos in the morning).

- Use a leave-in conditioner the night before. In the morning, use a little more or mist on a little water, which will reactivate the conditioner. It will enhance curls, smooth hair, or help add body and shine.

- Do NOT try a new hairstyle for picture day. Go with something you know looks good (and that you've already practiced and perfected on your kid).

- Choose a natural look rather than something fussy. Remember, it's your child's school picture, not her wedding photo!

- The hairstyle should be comfy for your kid . . . otherwise she will play around with it or pull it out.

- Your child should look like she normally does, so when you look back years later, the pic will seem real.

- For your older child, pack a small pocket brush or comb in case her hair needs a quick touch-up.

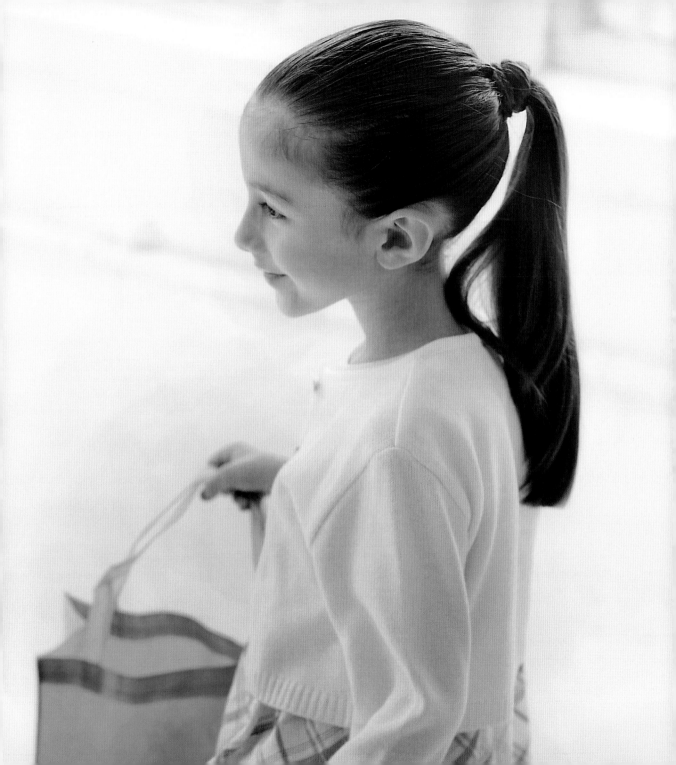

# Acknowledgments

It really is true that it takes a village! This book is the direct result of a tremendous team effort, and for that I would like to express my thanks and sincere gratitude to many people.

Sheryl Berk, for being a delight to work with, for going the extra mile when things got tough and for her incredible knowledge and passion for girls' hair, despite the fact that she isn't a hairstylist! Ingrid Abramovitch, for her vision, ideas, commitment to the project, and most especially her incredible patience when I was dealing with obstacles and unforeseen life events. Jill Cohen, for picking up the pieces! Jill is much more than a literary agent; her clear thinking and logical solutions kept this project intact. I'm appreciative that she took a chance on me, a first-time author. Thanks to Vincente Wolf for introducing us. Ann Bramson, for believing in this project, even when it got a little complicated. Katherine Camargo and Judy Pray, for their eagle eyes, keeping this book on the right track, and getting the best work out of us. Jan Derevjanik and Susan Baldaserini, for all the direction, suggestions, help, and experience that they generously shared. Thanks also to the rest of the Artisan team: Amy Corley, Barbara Peragine, Chrissa Yee, Erin Sainz, Jarrod Dyer, Nancy Murray, Suzanne Lander, and Trent Duffy.

The amazingly beautiful girls photographed in this book (and their parents) who generously volunteered their time and energy. I knew I was right to use "real" girls who are supermodels in my eyes: Allie Salerno, Allison Christine Lee, Amanda Irwin, Bailey Pollak, Becca Beal, Carly Geneen, Caroline Berk, Carson Riffkin, Charlotte Cohen, Ella Mansager, Hannah Samantha Levine, Hayley Schwartz, Jenna Ryan, Jordyn Cohen, Julia Gardner, Kate Salerno, Katherine Moses, Katherine Ohotin, Lola Simon, Lucy Mandel, Maddie Welton, Maggie Francis Levine, Maya Clark-Self, Noa Bella Garson, Nicole Radke, Rebecca Reich, Reina McNutt, Ruby Simon, Ryan Chisolm, Savanna Munroe, Spencer Jonas, Sofia Eleni Hrisitidis, Scarlet G. R. Walden, and Sparrow Gilligan.

The remarkable hairstylists from Cozy's Cuts For Kids who worked on the shoot: Cathy Desimone, Iris Deighan, Kristy Joy Danno, Marlena Feldman, and Tonia Lasaponara. I'm also thankful to all the stylists who worked behind the scenes planning, preparing, testing, and creating hairstyles, tips, and advice. I also want to thank all Cozy's stylists, even those who didn't work directly on this project, for the inspiration they have given to me: Annie Piazza-Sanchez, Berta Cuzo, Caroline Balza-Park, Christina Reinwald, Hope Pirpinias, Joaquin Martinez, Julia Korzun, Kimi Yang, Lana Botvinnik, Leslie Magno, Maria Rosa Ramos, Marian Schneider, Michele Stacy, Nancy O'Donnell, Neena Gomez, Pamela Noble, Patricia Savage, Stella Godosis, Valeria Arias, and Wendy Lopez. They all have the patience of saints, never-ending kindness, talent, and an enviable passion for the work that they do. I admire and appreciate them all.

The many people who are responsible for the smooth-running shoot, which was quite a feat! That includes all the people who not only participated directly, but prepared, scheduled, and coordinated the details. I cannot thank them enough: Adonis Williams, Judith Rice & Associates, Kathie Young, Lisa Campos, Fain Kolinsky, Peter Brucas, Sarah Alves, and Tamela Davis.

All the marvelous stores and companies that supplied us with the wonderful clothing, furniture, flowers, and accoutrements seen in this book: Alissa Company, Berkley Girl, Bow's Art, Catimini, Contemporary Headwear, Design Within Reach, Eli Zabar, Flowers by Zoe, Infinity, Lester's, Original Dr. Scholl's, The Pamela Company, Rachel Weissman, Ricky's NY, Seven For All Mankind, Splendid, and VW Home by Vincente Wolf.

Alexandra Grablewski, a photographic genius! What makes her photography so special is that she is able to capture a person's inner beauty in each shot. Todd Bonne, whose fun and easygoing style brought out the best in everyone and made the shoot seem like a party!

The experts who were so generous with their time, experience, and knowledge: Alan J. Bauman, MD, medical director, Bauman Medical Group; Gary Fishkin, CFN Beauty Representation; Jacob Guttman, Creative Styling Tools; Jen McDann, director of Cosmetology/Nail Technology, Tricoci University of Beauty Culture; Julia Youssef, VP Technical Center L'Oréal Paris; Jacqueline Beer, MD, FAD; James Crosty, Root Source Inc.; Michelle Breyer, NaturallyCurly.com; Marisa Fox Bevilacqua; Palmo Pasquariello, MD; and Ralf Zissel, Norman Research, LLC.

Fahima Ahmed, my right hand. Special thanks for keeping me organized and focused and for all the good judgment and insight; for holding down the fort when I couldn't and for never-ending support and loyalty. I'm so lucky to work with her.

My brother Alan, who has taught me to dream big and to think out of the box. I don't know what I would do without all his great advice and ideas.

Dad, Jackie, Danielle, and David—for all their love and confidence in me.

Marilyn and Marty Friedman, the greatest in-laws anyone could ever wish for. Thanks for all the millions of things they do for us and all their love and support.

My mom, an inspiration on every level. She didn't just give me life; she taught me how to live it.

Roberta Chevlowe, for her unwavering support and loyalty, going above and beyond the job of best friend. I'd also like to add a thank-you for all the years of sound legal advice (Tommy, too).

David Rogal, for being such a great friend and always being my last-minute savior ever since Mrs. Taylor's class.

Jill Sacher, the ultimate cheerleader and friend, who helped find me so many of the gorgeous girls in this book.

My husband Joey, who has taught me by example how to conquer adversity, with courage and determination, for inspiring me to run in the rain, and most importantly, for the never-ending support and love that he continues to give me unconditionally.

My amazing boys, Shane and Riley, who I adore and am so proud of.

There are so many others who have helped make this book possible, but not enough room to name them all. To those I haven't named, please know that I am very aware of their help, support, contributions and love—and I will always be grateful.

# *Index*